FREE Study Skills DVD Offer

Dear Customer,

Thank you for your purchase from Mometrix! We consider it an honor and privilege that you have purchased our product and want to ensure your satisfaction.

As a way of showing our appreciation and to help us better serve you, we have developed a Study Skills DVD that we would like to give you for <u>FREE</u>. **This DVD covers our "best practices" for studying for your exam, from using our study materials to preparing for the day of the test.**

All that we ask is that you email us your feedback that would describe your experience so far with our product. Good, bad or indifferent, we want to know what you think!

To get your **FREE Study Skills DVD**, email <u>freedvd@mometrix.com</u> with "FREE STUDY SKILLS DVD" in the subject line and the following information in the body of the email:

    a. The name of the product you purchased.

    b. Your product rating on a scale of 1-5, with 5 being the highest rating.

    c. Your feedback. It can be long, short, or anything in-between, just your impressions and experience so far with our product. Good feedback might include how our study material met your needs and will highlight features of the product that you found helpful.

    d. Your full name and shipping address where you would like us to send your free DVD.

If you have any questions or concerns, please don't hesitate to contact me directly.

Thanks again!

Sincerely,

Jay Willis
Vice President
<u>jay.willis@mometrix.com</u>
1-800-673-8175

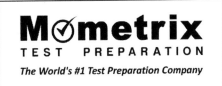

CHPN
Exam
SECRETS

Study Guide
Your Key to Exam Success

Unofficial CHPN Test Review for the
Certified Hospice and Palliative
Nurse Examination

Published by
Mometrix Test Preparation
CHPN Exam Secrets Test Prep Team

Written and edited by the CHPN Exam Secrets Test Prep Staff

Printed in the United States of America

This paper meets the requirements of ANSI/NISO Z39.48-1992 (Permanence of Paper).

Mometrix offers volume discount pricing to institutions. For more information or a price quote, please contact our sales department at sales@mometrix.com or 888-248-1219.

CHPN® is a registered trademark of Hospice and Palliative Credentialing Center (HPCC), which was not involved in the production of, and does not endorse, this product.

ISBN 13: 978-1-60971-344-7
ISBN 10: 1-60971-344-3

Dear Future Exam Success Story:

Congratulations on your purchase of our study guide. Our goal in writing our study guide was to cover the content on the test, as well as provide insight into typical test taking mistakes and how to overcome them.

Standardized tests are a key component of being successful, which only increases the importance of doing well in the high-pressure high-stakes environment of test day. How well you do on this test will have a significant impact on your future- and we have the research and practical advice to help you execute on test day.

The product you're reading now is designed to exploit weaknesses in the test itself, and help you avoid the most common errors test takers frequently make.

How to use this study guide

We don't want to waste your time. Our study guide is fast-paced and fluff-free. We suggest going through it a number of times, as repetition is an important part of learning new information and concepts.

First, read through the study guide completely to get a feel for the content and organization. Read the general success strategies first, and then proceed to the content sections. Each tip has been carefully selected for its effectiveness.

Second, read through the study guide again, and take notes in the margins and highlight those sections where you may have a particular weakness.

Finally, bring the manual with you on test day and study it before the exam begins.

Your success is our success

We would be delighted to hear about your success. Send us an email and tell us your story. Thanks for your business and we wish you continued success-

Sincerely,

Mometrix Test Preparation Team

Need more help? Check out our flashcards at: http://MometrixFlashcards.com/NBCHPN

TABLE OF CONTENTS

Top 20 Test Taking Tips

1. Carefully follow all the test registration procedures
2. Know the test directions, duration, topics, question types, how many questions
3. Setup a flexible study schedule at least 3-4 weeks before test day
4. Study during the time of day you are most alert, relaxed, and stress free
5. Maximize your learning style; visual learner use visual study aids, auditory learner use auditory study aids
6. Focus on your weakest knowledge base
7. Find a study partner to review with and help clarify questions
8. Practice, practice, practice
9. Get a good night's sleep; don't try to cram the night before the test
10. Eat a well balanced meal
11. Know the exact physical location of the testing site; drive the route to the site prior to test day
12. Bring a set of ear plugs; the testing center could be noisy
13. Wear comfortable, loose fitting, layered clothing to the testing center; prepare for it to be either cold or hot during the test
14. Bring at least 2 current forms of ID to the testing center
15. Arrive to the test early; be prepared to wait and be patient
16. Eliminate the obviously wrong answer choices, then guess the first remaining choice
17. Pace yourself; don't rush, but keep working and move on if you get stuck
18. Maintain a positive attitude even if the test is going poorly
19. Keep your first answer unless you are positive it is wrong
20. Check your work, don't make a careless mistake

Patient and Family Care, Education, and Advocacy

Suffering

There are multiple aspects of suffering in which an individual can feel pain or distress; it encompasses emotional, spiritual, and physical aspects of life and affects the whole person. Suffering must be addressed from a comprehensive, holistic perspective while recognizing that it is not always possible to find the source, or resolve, suffering. Identification of suffering involves careful observation and different disciplinary perspectives can be helpful in making an accurate assessment. Issues surrounding suffering must be addressed or the suffering is more likely to compound rather than diminish over time. However, when the patient addresses these questions it is not necessarily expected for the caregiver to give, or have, the answers to the questions. Rather, the caregiver should reassure the patient of his or her presence and support while patients explore these questions and find answers for themselves. Religious or spiritual counseling and exploration is often useful as well.

Collaborating with patient and family to identify goals and outcomes

When collaborating with the patient and family, the hospital and palliative care nurse should begin by educating the patient and family about patient rights and asking what outcomes they desire. In order to develop the plan of care, the nurse must know what the patient and family desire in terms of goals and outcomes. For example, if a patient's goal is to remain mentally alert until death, this may affect the plan for managing pain. If a desired outcome is that the patient die in the home, then the plan of care must include the resources needed to facilitate this. The nurse should ask that the patient and caregiver or other family members list the goals and outcomes that are most important to them and then should compare and discuss the items as they may not always be in agreement and some negotiation and discussion may be required. While a patient may want to remain at home, for example, the caregiver may prefer that the patient be hospitalized.

Developing a care path

The following is the six-step process for developing a care path:
1. Identify cases that are statistically significant and carry a high priority. Review medical records and research credible literature related to the specific problem. Evaluate the specific characteristics of the problem regarding symptoms, average length of hospital stay, critical or life-threatening factors, and positive outcomes.
2. Record the critical path, sequencing, and timing of the appropriate functions to be implemented by all health care providers.
3. Recruit nurses, physicians, and other disciplines to become involved in the review process for the plan of care.
4. Make revisions to the pathway as needed until a group consensus has been reached for the key care components.
5. Implement the pathway and evaluate for additional revisions.
6. Expand the implementation of the pathway of patient management into quality-improvement programs. Continue to monitor and evaluate patient-based outcomes.

Successful palliative care program

The following are elements of a successful palliative care program:
- A well-defined vision and mission for quality palliative care.
- Effective implementation strategies that consider both human needs and available resources.
- Support and advocating efforts by all team members for quality palliative care.
- Learn from and coordinate effectively with acute care settings.
- Continual quality improvement: finding ways to effectively deliver the "right" care easily and efficiently.
- Dynamic education processes and support of innovative programs.
- Increased autonomy and authority of palliative care team members.
- Attention to and respect for cultural and ethnic diversity.
- Focused efforts to improve access to and the quality of palliative care, the effective use of resources, and greater patient and family satisfaction.
- Effective communication on all levels of the program, including community stakeholders.

Hospice and palliative care in the United States

The Connecticut Hospice was founded by Florence Wald (former Dean of the Yale Nursing School) in the early 1970s. It was modeled after the work of Dame Cicely Saunders at the St. Christopher's Hospice in London, England. These hospice programs were developed to address the specific needs of the dying and their families. Hospice care became a Medicare/Medicaid benefit in the 1980s. The palliative care model branched off from traditional hospice programs in the late 1980s in academic teaching hospitals such as the Cleveland Clinic and Medical College of Wisconsin. The palliative focus was to address problems facing the hospice philosophy in addressing long-term, progressive disease paths as well as in allowing patients a choice of therapies. An effort was also made to improve the quality-of-life concerns for those patients whose death was not near yet, a distinct and complicated set of care issues. Palliative care is not regulated or funded by Medicare.

Hospice interdimensional care process

The five steps in the hospice interdimensional care process are:
1. Perform an in depth, holistic assessment in order to collect both subjective and objective data from the patient and family.
2. Root cause for needs, problems, and opportunities to improve the patient's quality of life. These identified problems and needs become the backbone for all care provided.
3. Collaborate with the interdisciplinary team members to set patient- and family-directed goals and establish appropriate interventions. These goals and interventions should be mutually understood and accepted by all team members.
4. Provide palliative therapeutic care, education, collaboration, and ongoing assessments that empower the patient and family and focus on their needs.
5. Evaluate all care and interventions for future planning, identifying productive areas for continuation and areas needing revision.

Hospice

Hospice care is designed to fit the needs of terminally ill in the last 6 months of life. Hospice is founded on a philosophy of improved quality of life for the terminally ill. It offers symptom management, physical care, emotional care, psychosocial care, spiritual care, and bereavement care. This care may be provided in many settings, including inpatient settings and various residential settings. The overall focus is to provide comfort and support to patients and their families experiencing a life-limiting illness when cure-oriented treatments are no longer feasible. Hospice caregivers offer a specialized knowledge of medical care and symptom management, with special emphasis on pain and discomfort management. Hospice is not designed to either prolong life or hasten the death of the individual but rather improve the quality of the patient's last days through comfort and dignity.

Possible adaptations in hospice or palliative care

Adaptations needed in the environment may vary widely for the hospice or palliative care patient:
- Access issues: If the patient needs to use a wheelchair, furniture may need to be moved, doorways widened, and/or a wheelchair ramp installed. If the bathroom is difficult to access (upstairs, not wheelchair accessible), a bedside commode may be needed. Items may need to be moved or placed so they are easier to reach.
- Safety issues: Grab bars may need to be installed in bathrooms, hallways, and stairways and scatter rugs removed. Lighting may need to be improved. Patients may need assistive devices, such as wheelchairs, canes, and walkers. If patients are confused/disoriented/wandering, the home may need door latches, movement alarms, and other safety devices.
- Equipment issues: The patient may need a hospital bed or other equipment to facilitate care or relieve symptoms, and this can involve changes in wiring, moving furniture, and sometimes changing rooms.

Services provided under the Medicare Hospice Model

Hospice units under this model provide care within the eligibility and funding available through the Medicare regulations. Core services that maintain the general health and quality of life for the patient, such as physician and nursing services, social work, dietary services, spiritual, and bereavement counseling, are required by law and provided at the Medicare level of care. Further services may be added based on patient need and availability. These added benefits may include physical, occupational, speech, massage, and infusion therapy. Home health aides and medical supplies and equipment are also common. Daycare and homemaking services, as well as funeral services, may also be offered as needed for support of the patient and family at this level.

Eligibility requirements for hospice and palliative care

Hospice eligibility is directly related to the patient's prognosis. To receive hospice services, it is expected that the patient will reach the end of life through the course of the natural disease process within 6 months of qualifying. Certification from the physician confirming this status is required and can limit access for some who may have benefited. Education is still needed to reinforce to physicians the timely referral of patients. Eligibility for palliative care exceeds 6 months and is designed to meet the needs of a variety of individuals with chronic illnesses such as Alzheimer disease. It is not limited to comfort care or a specific time frame. Any treatment the patient and family desire as a means to improve the quality of life is respected by the palliative care team. Cost aspects must also be considered; however, hospice funding is available for those who qualify for Medicare and Medicaid. This is not the case with palliative care.

Community resources for hospice or palliative care patients

Community resources that may be helpful for the hospice or palliative care patient include:
- Home health agencies: These can provide homebound patients with medical treatment, monitoring, and personal care (bathing) and referral to other needed services, such as a social worker.
- Volunteer agencies: These vary but may include faith-based or other volunteers who will visit, assist with shopping and/or cooking, transport patients, sit with patients, or carry out other non-skilled activities to support the patient and family.
- Medical supply companies: Patients may need a wide variety of assistive devices, including small items such as grab/reach tools, tub rails, and grab bars, and larger devices, such as wheelchairs, walkers, lifts, and hospital beds.
- Educational resources: These may include libraries (medical and general), podcasts, videos, national organizations (such as the Alzheimer's Association), and Internet sources.
- Support groups: Local hospitals, senior centers, and organizations often provide a variety of support groups for both patients and family/caregivers, such as support groups for those with cancer.
- Meal programs: Home meal delivery may be necessary.

Palliative care

Palliative care begins by recognizing and respecting each individual's uniqueness across the lifespan and in diverse settings. It is patient-centered and guided in order to improve the patient's quality of life through supportive care. It is both scientific and humanistic. Palliative care does not limit the patient's treatment options and includes any therapy medically indicated and desired by the patient. This includes life-prolonging care even when death is imminent. The World Health Organization defines palliative care as "an approach that improves quality of life of patients and their families facing the problem associated with life-threatening illness, through the prevention and relief of suffering by means of early identification and impeccable assessment and treatment of pain and other problems, physical, psychosocial and spiritual." Effective palliative care includes multiple dimensions of care, including a holistic approach to pain and symptom control, nursing interventions, and psychosocial and spiritual resources to provide an active, caring presence for patients and families.

Family-centered palliative care

Family-centered care is a fundamental principle in the palliative care philosophy. This philosophy recognizes the terminally ill patient's place within a family environment. The illness, in turn, has an effect on the entire family, necessitating the involvement of the whole family in the plan of care. The nurse must coordinate and plan care based not only on the individual needs of the patient, but on the needs of the patient as a family member and the needs of additional family members as well. How the patient functions within the family unit is a vital portion of the patient's needs in a transitioning life structure. This transition is experienced by the entire family and each member will play a role in the loss experience.

Health problems associated with poverty and homelessness

Individuals who are poor or homeless are restricted in their access to health care and more likely to die from cancer and other diseases than other individuals. Education and outreach programs are often inappropriate or irrelevant in their lives; they foster a sense of fatalism concerning their health. Health risks for the poor and homeless can be classified into the following categories:

- Malnutrition and wasting.
- A lack of shelter and access to bathing facilities, leading to skin infections, lice, cellulites, podiatric problems, hypothermia, tuberculosis, and dental problems.
- Drug and alcohol use causing overdose, seizures, delirium, sexually transmitted infections, trauma from falls or other accidents, cirrhosis, heroin nephropathy, or esophageal varices.
- Chronic mental illnesses, such as paranoid ideation, antisocial behaviors, psychosis, and suicide.
- Violence-related injuries, such as assaults, homicides, and rape.

Risk factors for medication use in the elderly

Multiple health care professionals such as physicians and practitioners can be involved in providing care for elderly patients. This situation can lead to multiple medication prescriptions, sometimes conflicting with each other. Multiple prescriptions can also lead to complex dosing schedules, route, or parameters for medication delivery. Other age-related factors can also contribute to medication risks. Age-related physiological pharmacokinetic and pharmacodynamic changes can take place. In the presence of visual and hearing difficulties, confusion about indications and medication regimens can easily happen. Cognitive changes such as delirium, dementia, depression, and anxiety can also lead to medication errors. The individual may also be self-medicating with over-the-counter medications, alcohol, or herbal remedies, a situation which may be unknown to the health care provider. Miscellaneous factors can also include the lack of social support, finances, fears of addiction or side effects, and language barriers.

Disposition of schedule II drugs in patient's home after death

By law, Schedule II drugs should be discarded by the nurse or medical professional who is responsible for medication management at the time of death of a patient. This medication waste needs to occur as soon after the death as reasonable and needs to be witnessed and verified by a second qualified individual. The drugs have been paid for as part of the patient's care, so they do not belong to the hospice or palliative care program. Medications cannot be returned to useful pharmacy stock because there is no guarantee that the medications have not been altered.

Cultural competence

Culturally competent behavior goes beyond knowing general facts; it is a dynamic process of being aware of and showing respect for cultural differences of all types. It begins with being aware of one's own beliefs and not letting them interfere with the care provided. Just as each nurse brings his or her own individual background, beliefs, and practices to the caring experience, each patient and family have their own unique contributions to the care plan. Cultural competence is providing competent care that corresponds with the patient and family's own cultural background. The nurse provides a complete and unbiased, sensitive assessment of the patient's background and beliefs, obtains further knowledge as necessary, then coordinates and executes a plan of care that is meaningful to the patient and family, regardless of the care provider's own beliefs.

Respecting patients from diverse cultures

Each person is entitled to receive an individualized full assessment and personal care. The nurse should first assess his/her own background, values, and beliefs in order to consciously avoid biases. Obtain further knowledge in order to understand the background being addressed and to show acceptance of differences even when they may diverge from the nurse's own comfort zone and culture. Acknowledge differences concerning end-of-life care, be sensitive, and be open to the individual patient's beliefs rather than trying to predict behavior. Assumptions regarding care, needs, or beliefs should not be made based on race or ethnicity.

Spiritual care of hospice patient and family

The patient's basic beliefs should be assessed in order to provide holistic care at the end of life. Spiritual care must be provided according to the patient's religion of choice, and the caregiver must be unbiased regardless of his or her own beliefs. If patients do not wish to have spiritual counseling, it should not be forced on them. Advice and comfort can be provided by anyone known to the patient. It is intended to relieve spiritual suffering and answer questions the patient and family may have. Even those who do not have a formal religion or practice may have questions and search for meaning and comfort at the end of life.

Complete spiritual assessment

The caregiver must assess prior and present religious affiliations and beliefs about God and the afterlife. Information must include devotional practices, rituals, and routines, and identify the degree of involvement and support available from the patient's chosen religious community. This spiritual assessment opens the door for effective spiritual caregiving; it allows patients and their families to access spiritual coping strategies and support mechanisms. The holistic assessment addresses the patient's ability to resolve meaningful spiritual questions, identifying meaning and retaining hope, strength, and peace. Questions can include the patient's interpretation of the meaning and purpose of their life, personal strengths, and connections to various spiritual communities including nature. Provisions should be made to explore spiritual relationships and provide support for loss and crisis as desired by the patient and family.

HOPE and FICA

HOPE is a simple mnemonic used as a guideline for the spiritual assessment.
- H – Hope: What sources of hope (who or what) do you have to turn to?
- – Organized: Are you a part of an organized religion or faith group? What do you gain from membership in this group?
- P – Personal: What personal spiritual practices such as prayer or meditation are most helpful to you?
- E – Effects: What effects do your beliefs play on any medical care or end-of-life issues and decisions? Do you have any beliefs that may affect the type of care the health care team can provide you with?

FICA is another abbreviated spiritual assessment tool.
- F – Faith: Do you have a faith or belief system that gives your life meaning?
- I – Importance: What significance does your faith have in your daily life?
- C – Community: Do you participate and gain support from a faith community?
- A – Address: What faith issues would you like me to address in your care?

SPIRIT

SPIRIT is a mnemonic used for a spiritual assessment tool:
- S – Spiritual: Do you have a formal religious affiliation?
- P – Personal: Which practices and beliefs do you personally accept and practice? Does spirituality play a part in your daily life?
- I – Integration: Do you participate in a spiritual community and receive support from that community?
- R – Ritual: Are there specific practices and restrictions in your religious convictions that would affect your health care choices?
- I – Implication: Are there aspects of your spirituality you would like me to keep in mind during your care?
- T – Terminal Events: As you prepare for the end-of-life, how does your faith affect the decisions you make or how you feel about death?

Communication in palliative care

A vital role of the nurse in a palliative care setting is to facilitate communication and establish a trusting relationship with the patient and family. Communication takes place on many different levels and the message received may not always be in control of the sender. In fact, as much as 80% of all communication takes place nonverbally. Though the information can be overwhelming to the patient or family, most individuals expect honesty and truthfulness in their communications with the health care provider. Communication should establish trust and openness, include the patient and family in all options and care decisions, assure the individual that they will be listened to and respected (that they will not be ignored or abandoned), avoid and resolve conflict, and allow patients to vocalize their needs and expect them to be addressed. It is also important to extend this communication to the entire health care team to facilitate understanding and continuity of care.

Overcoming language barriers

Health care agencies that are federally funded are required to provide free interpretive services for clients speaking commonly encountered foreign languages. The patient must be informed that an interpreter will be made available to them. In order to ensure appropriate care and communication, a third party interpreter who is trained in medical terminology, fluent in both languages being used, and familiar with the ethics and HIPAA regulations of acting as an interpreter is the best option. Meeting these requirements ensures compliance with federal guidelines. Family members cannot be required to serve as interpreters unless the client specifically requests a family member to act in this capacity. In emergency situations, it is appropriate to use whatever means are readily available to assist in communicating with the patient.

Establishing and maintaining therapeutic relationships

Therapeutic relationships are established on principles of empathy, unconditional positive regard, and genuineness. To build these qualities, the nurse must express empathy (try to understand the individual's viewpoint), nonjudgmental acceptance of the other individual, genuine concern and respect, and an attention to detail. The nurse should have the ability to convey trustworthiness, honesty, and openness in a professional manner. An attention to detail allows the nurse to think critically and analyze a situation without drawing hasty conclusions or assumptions. The nurse tries to be attentive to his or her own part in the relationship, watching for actions, words, or attitudes that may be destructive to the relationship if they are misinterpreted by the other party.

Attentive listening

Attentive listeners are actively trying to understand and remember the messages they are hearing. They use appropriate nonverbal signals and body language, such as facing the speaker directly, maintaining an open posture and appropriate distance for patient comfort, making no unnecessary body movements, using appropriate facial expression, and maintaining eye contact with the other person. They demonstrate interest in what is being said by showing respect for the speaker, not interrupting the speaker, maintaining attention to the conversation and avoiding multitasking, encouraging dialogue and discussion, asking appropriate questions, and providing an unhurried and comfortable environment with minimal distractions for communication. Attentive listeners also affirm the speaker and message by nodding, providing occasional, nonjudgmental summaries of what has been said, asking for clarifications when needed, and reflecting the mood and message being communicated appropriately in their expression and body language.

Guidelines for delivering unfavorable or bad news

Girgis and Sanson-Fisher recommend the following eight steps as guidelines a caregiver can use when delivering unfavorable or bad news.
1. Provide privacy and adequate time. Create a setting that is quiet and comfortable where participants will feel unrushed and uninterrupted. Establish who should be present.
2. Assess understanding. Be informed about the condition. Determine what the family and patient already know.
3. Provide information simply and honestly. Give a warning and allow participants to prepare themselves for the discussion. Clearly express the goals of the meeting. Establish a foundation of basic information that can be built upon. Use common language and easy to understand explanations. Provide an interpreter if necessary.
4. Avoid euphemisms. Discuss matters in a clear and direct manner.
5. Encourage the expression of feelings. Confirm and accept all emotional responses.
6. Be empathetic. Sit quietly and allow time for information to be absorbed. Listen carefully and refrain from judgment.
7. Give a broad, but realistic, time frame for disease progression. Allow for questions and comments. Discuss the need for a legal decision maker. Watch for indications of self-harm intentions.
8. Arrange for a review or follow up.

Maintaining a sense of hope in terminally ill patients

Multiple factors can affect the individual's outlook during a terminal illness. These include the ability to experience one or more meaningful relationships. The individual needs to feel a sense of

- 9 -

being needed, a part of something. Maintaining feelings of lightheartedness, delight, joy, or playfulness helps the individual identify positive personal attributes. They are more accepting of themselves and others as they continue to be able to identify courage, determination, serenity, and positive self-worth. Spiritual beliefs and participation in spiritual rituals provide a sense of meaning to their lives. The individual can focus their energy on achieving short-term, positive goals that provide direction to their lives and allow them to continue to share themselves with others. In the final stages of a terminal illness, individuals who have maintained a feeling of hope are able to look toward their eventual death with peace and serenity.

Identifying unrealistic hope

In assessing whether the hope an individual is experiencing is unrealistic, determine if the hope is broad or too severe, such as complete denial of the disease process or belief of a cure when there is none available. If the hope is unlikely to be realized, how determined is the individual to their course? Is he or she able to admit at times that there are limitations and acknowledge the possibility of a negative outcome? Does the individual state he or she has a sure knowledge of what will happen rather than expressing realistic hopes and fears? Those experiencing unrealistic hope are more likely to engage in reckless behaviors and ignore or avoid acknowledging worsening symptoms or warning signs. This unrealistic hope may alienate the individual from family and friends, creating isolation. Is the person experiencing increased distress and anxiety? Is he or she impeding his or her ability to place personal affairs in order or acknowledge their own loss?

Maladaptive behaviors of patients and families

The following are 6 maladaptive behaviors patients and families dealing with life-threatening illnesses may use:
- Denial: Denial is a way for the person to reject the reality of the situation they find themselves in. It is a refusal of physical, psychological, and emotional triggers of knowledge they do not want to believe or deal with.
- Guilt: An unreasonable feeling of responsibility for negative influences of which the person may or may not have control.
- Depression: A mental state of hopelessness and despair. A severe loss of happiness and motivation.
- Avoidance: Withdrawal; turning away from actions or consequences associated with negative stimulus.
- Decathexis: Detachment from mood and feelings; a lack of variation in emotional responses despite changing circumstances.
- Aggression: Hostile behavior, physical or verbal, meant to be demeaning, destructive, and increase negative emotions in those around them.

Grief

Grief is an emotional response to a loss that begins at the time a loss is anticipated and continues on an individual timetable. While there are identifiable stages or tasks, is not an orderly and predictable process. It involves overcoming anger, disbelief, guilt, and a myriad of related emotions. The grieving individual may move back and forth between stages or experience several emotions at any given time. Each person's grief response is unique to their own coping patterns, stress levels, age, gender, belief system, and previous experiences with loss.

Anticipatory grief

Anticipatory grief is the mental, social, and somatic reactions of an individual as they prepare themselves for a perceived future loss. The individual experiences a process of intellectual, emotional, and behavioral responses in order to modify their self-concept, based on their perception of what the potential loss will mean in their life. This process often takes place ahead of the actual loss, from the time the loss is first perceived until it is resolved as a reality for the individual. This process can also blend with past loss experiences. It is associated with the individual's perception of how life will be affected by the particular diagnosis as well as the impending death. Acknowledging this anticipatory grief allows family members to begin looking toward a changed future. Suppressing this anticipatory process may inhibit relationships with the ill individual and contribute to a more difficult grieving process at a later time. However, appropriate anticipatory grieving does not take the place of grief during the actual time of death.

Disenfranchised grief

Disenfranchised grief occurs when the loss being experienced cannot be openly acknowledged, publicly mourned, or socially supported. Society and culture are partly responsible for an individual's response to a loss. There is a social context to grief; if a person incurring the loss will be putting himself or herself at risk if grief is expressed, disenfranchised grief occurs. The risk for disenfranchised grief is greatest among those whose relationship with the individual they lost was not known or regarded as significant. This is also the situation found among bereaved persons who are not recognized by society as capable of grief, such as young children, or needing to mourn, such as an ex-spouse or secret lover.

Grief and depression

Normal grief is preoccupied with self-limiting to the loss itself. Emotional responses will vary and may include open expressions of anger. The individual may experience difficulty sleeping or vivid dreams, a lack of energy, and weight loss. Crying is evident and provides some relief of extreme emotions. The individual remains socially responsive and seeks reassurance from others.

Depression is marked by extensive periods of sadness and preoccupation often extending beyond 2 months. It is not limited to the single event. There is an absence of pleasure or anger and isolation from previous social support systems. The individual can experience extreme lethargy, weight loss, insomnia, or hypersomnia, and has no recollection of dreaming. Crying is absent or persistent and provides no relief of emotions. Professional intervention is required to relieve depression.

Loss

Loss is the blanket term used to denote the absence of a valued object, position, ability, attribute, or individual. The aspect of loss as it is associated with the death of an animal or person is a relatively new definition. Loss is an individualized and subjective experience depending on the perceived attachment between the individual and the missing aspect. This can range from little or no value of attachment to significant value. Loss also can be represented by the withdrawal of a valued relationship one had or would have had in the future. Depending on the unique and individual responses to the perception of loss and its significance, reactions to the loss with vary accordingly. Robinson and McKenna summarize the aspects of loss in three main attributes:
- Something has been removed.
- The item removed had value to that person.
- The response is individualized

Mourning

Mourning is a public grief response for the death of a loved one. The various aspects of the mourning process are partially determined by personal and cultural belief systems. Kagawa-Singer defines mourning as "the social customs and cultural practices that follow a death." Durkheim expands this to include the following: "mourning is not a natural movement of private feelings wounded by a cruel loss; it is a duty imposed by the group." Mourning involves participation in religious and culturally appropriate customs and rituals designed to publicly acknowledge the loss. These rituals signify they are adjusting to the change in their relationships created by the loss, as well as mark the beginning of the reorganization and forward movement of their lives.

Bereavement

Bereavement is the emotional and mental state associated with having suffered a personal loss. It is the reactions of grief and sadness initiated by the loss of a loved one. Bereavement is a normal process of feeling deprived of something of value. The word bereave comes from the root "reave" meaning to plunder, spoil, or rob. It is recognized that the lost individual had value and a defining role in the surviving individual's life. Bereavement encompasses all the acts and emotions surrounding the feeling of loss for the individual. During this grieving period, there is an increased mortality risk. A positive bereavement experience means being able to recognize the significance of the loss while still recognizing the resilience and value of life.

Factors complicating bereavement
The caregiver should assess for multiple life crises that take energy away from the grieving process. An important factor is the grieving individual's history with past grieving experiences. Assess for other recent, unresolved, or difficult losses that may need to be addressed before the individual can move toward resolution of the current loss. Age, mental health, substance abuse, extreme anger, anxiety, or dependence on the individual facing the end of life can add additional stressors and handicap natural coping mechanisms. Income strains, community support, outside and personal responsibilities, the absence of cultural and religious beliefs, the difficulty of the disease process, and age of the loved one lost can also present additional risk factors.

Coping with dying

The following is the task-based model for coping with dying:
- Physical tasks: Bodily needs must be met and physical distress minimized in ways that are consistent with the patient's values and beliefs.
- Psychological tasks: The patient must feel a sense of dignity. They seek reassurance and satisfaction in their lives, security, and autonomy.
- Social tasks: Seeking to resolve and sustain interpersonal relationships that are significant to them and to address social implications of dying.
- Spiritual tasks: Identify, develop, and reaffirm sources of spiritual energy and comfort in order to define the purpose to their existence and create hope.

Fears of dying patients

Common fears of dying patients are as follows:
- Pain: Patients commonly fear lingering and uncontrolled suffering. Relieving discomfort provides improved quality of life.
- Fear of being a burden: Patient's family and friends face the tasks of dealing with their own fears as well as increased responsibility for the patient that can be taxing and unwelcome by either party.
- Fear of loss of control and independence: Patients need to maintain a sense of control in decision-making in all areas of their life and care. A sense of control helps alleviate feelings of guilt, frustration, and helplessness during illness.
- Fear of dying alone: Ill persons often feel they will be abandoned.
- Death: Patients who are unsettled in their beliefs about an afterlife are facing the unknown. They may also fear leaving loved ones or "unfinished business."
- Bodily changes: Loss of body parts and changes to physique can be unnerving and shift the patient's sense of self.

Rights of newborn and infants in palliative care

The newborn or infant maintains the right to be listened to as an individual person with rights. The infant is not the property of his or her parents, caregivers, medical personnel, or society. An infant has the right to cry as a natural course of their emotions. These cries should be acknowledged and comfort given as it is needed. He or she can create fantasies. An infant is still capable of, and entitled to, hope. The infant or newborn should not be restricted from interacting with his or her siblings and parents. Their needs can be met at home or in the hospital, wherever their parents are comfortable having that care delivered. In either situation, family members may help provide that care.

Care of the body

The body should be prepared to give a clean, peaceful impression for those family members who desire an opportunity to say goodbye before funeral home removal. Kindly caring for the body shows the family care and concern and the continued value of the deceased, as well as models grief-facilitating behaviors for others present. Religious or other rituals the family may find comforting should be encouraged, as well as inviting them to participate in the preparation of the body. Explain the process and what to expect as care is given. Unless otherwise indicated by protocol or the need for autopsy, any tubes, drains, and other medical devices should be removed. Bandages should be applied as fluids may still be expressed. A waterproof pad or incontinence brief underneath the body is helpful for containing fluids. Packing of the vagina or rectum is unnecessary. Wash the body and comb the hair. Consider dressing the body in something normalizing. It should be noted that the body may "sigh" as it is rolled and the lungs are compressed. If the area is kept cool, the decomposition process will be slowed, allowing the family time to grieve.

Postmortem decomposition

The bruising and softening of the body are largely related to the breakdown of red blood cells. As the cells breakdown, hemoglobin is released, resulting in a staining effect on the vessel walls and surrounding tissues. This mottling or bruising most frequently appears on dependent parts of the body as well as any areas that experienced recent trauma, such as puncture wounds from invasive procedures. The discoloration can become extensive in a very short period of time. The remainder of the body takes on a gray hue. The face often appears purple in color when death is the result of cardiac complications. The nurse should assure family members that this bruising process is a normal after-death occurrence.

Algor Mortis

When circulation and the hypothalamus stop functioning, the body's core temperature begins to drop by about 1.8 degrees every hour until it reaches a stasis at room temperature. The skin begins to lose its natural elasticity as the body cools. If a high fever was present at the time of death, the person may lose excess fluid through the skin, causing the skin to feel moist or giving the appearance of sweating even after death. This loss of moisture and elasticity causes the skin to become more fragile and easily damaged. The body should be handled gently, avoiding excess pressure or traction on the skin. Dressings should be applied with a wrap or paper tape.

Quality end-of-life

Quality end-of-life care should be initiated when supportive care and quality of life become the primary patient and family concerns. Each patient and family should experience continuity in quality of care with standardized protocols and measurable outcomes. The best medical treatment should be provided to improve patient function where possible. The patient should be free from overwhelming pain and other distressing symptoms as much as possible. Comfort should be ensured always. Health care should be continuous, comprehensive, and coordinated. In quality end-of-life care, the patient and family feel prepared for future events and understand what is likely to happen over the course of the illness. Patients and families should feel respected and valued, having their wishes sought, appreciated, and followed as much as possible. High-quality end-of-life care allows the patient to have dignity, self-respect, and the ability to make the best of every day, while having a sense of control. The patient's burden is relieved and relationships are strengthened.

Rigor Mortis

Within 4 hours of death, adenosine phosphate (ATP) is no longer synthesized because of the depletion of glycogen stores. ATP affects muscle fiber relaxation; the resulting lack of ATP causes an exaggerated contraction of the muscle fibers and immobilizes the joints. Rigor begins in the involuntary muscles found in the heart, gastrointestinal tract, bladder, and arteries. It then progresses through the muscles of the head, neck, trunk, and lower limbs. However, after approximately 96 hours the muscle activity totally ceases. The rigor passes. Those with large muscle mass may be prone to more pronounced rigor mortis. On the other hand, frail individuals are less prone toward to rigor mortis. Post-death positioning to minimize the effects of rigor mortis should include being sure the limbs and hands are in proper body alignment. Eyelids and jaw should be closed and dentures should be in place in the mouth.

Necessary documentation at time of death

Commonly, the patient is identified and then assessed for general appearance, lack of reflex or response to stimulus, including pupils that are fixed and dilated, the absence of breathing and lung sound, and the absence of both apical and carotid pulse. Documentation should include the patient's name and time of contact and death pronunciation, as well as who was present at the time of death, including health care personnel, family members, and friends. The time of the assessment, details of the physical examination, time the physician assessed the patient or was notified, and identification

- 14 -

of all parties notified of the death should be documented. Special plans for disposition, including organ donation, autopsy, and cultural or religious procedures, should also be noted.

Death pronouncement

Prior to the time of death, a plan should be in place for who will be contacted when death occurs, regardless of the location. Procedures for death pronouncement vary between state to state and sometimes within the individual state as well. Whether nurses can pronounce death is determined by the state. If the death occurs within an inpatient setting, organizational policy should be followed. In general, when a death occurs in a hospice setting, the nurse makes a visit for patient assessment, and then verbally conveys the absence of vital signs and other pertinent information to the physician for confirmation. The nurse then contacts the funeral home or mortuary. It may be necessary to also contact the police or coroner if the circumstances of the death were unusual, associated with a traumatic event, or occurred within 24 hours of a hospital admission.

Assessing caregiver ability

Assessing caregiver ability begins with asking the caregiver about the skills the person has, what the caregiver feels comfortable doing, and what areas the caregiver needs assistance. This shows respect for the caregiver and allows the caregiver to express concerns. The best method of assessing the actual skills is to work with the caregiver and observe, providing positive feedback during the process. Rather than criticizing, "Don't pull your spouse under the arms," a better approach is focus on the caregiver's needs, "Let me show you how to move your spouse without risking injuring your back." Assessment should include not only the caregiver's knowledge and physical ability to provide care but also the caregiver's emotional ability, resources available, values, and perceptions. It's important to know if the caregiver is willing to provide care or is doing so out of necessity, as this may affect the caregiver's sense of wellbeing and the patient-caregiver relationship.

Responding to caregiver fatigue

Caregiver fatigue is very common and can relate to physical or emotional fatigue. The hospice and palliative care nurse should discuss issues of caregiver fatigue early in the care process, if possible, so that the caregiver is aware of the effects of stress and overwork. Caregivers often get inadequate sleep and become exhausted from the constant demands of patient care and may not know where to turn for help. The nurse should address signs of fatigue directly, "You look exhausted," to encourage the caregiver to discuss problems. If the patient is under hospice care and is eligible for respite care, the nurse can help to facilitate a respite stay. The nurse can assess the environment to determine if accommodations would be helpful, and then provide the caregiver with information about community resources that may reduce the burden of care, such as Meals-on-Wheels, volunteers, adult day care, and caregiver support groups.

Principles of adult learning

Malcolm Knowles, the pioneer of adult learning, identifies the following characteristics of an adult learner.
- Adult learners are autonomous and self-directed and should be shown respect. They need to be actively involved in the learning process and empowered in the learning experience.
- Each adult has unique life experiences and knowledge that he or she brings to the learning experience, which can be drawn upon to assimilate new knowledge. Adult learners also demonstrate critical thinking abilities.
- Adults are generally goal-oriented. They must understand the value behind what is to be learned. They are also relevancy-oriented. The goal of the learning experience must have personal value to them.
- Adults are practical and want to focus their learning on those things that will be of most use.

Effects of anxiety on learning

Mild anxiety can facilitate learning by enhancing awareness and promoting information-seeking behaviors. The individual is able to absorb, process, and test new information within their personal parameters. Moderate anxiety begins to narrow the perceptual field but the individual can still be directed to observe and learn from new information. Severe anxiety greatly reduces the individual's ability to absorb new information because the person's focus is on providing immediate relief. Automatic, distancing, or self-soothing behaviors may be initiated in an attempt to re-establish equilibrium. Uncontrolled, severe anxiety can give way to feelings of panic, awe, or dread. Information is scattered and misinterpreted. There is an inability to focus attention outside of themselves or immediate needs. Control must be re-established before learning can take place.

Fentanyl patch

The fentanyl patch should be placed on a clean, dry, hairless portion of the upper body; it is absorbed better when placed over some adipose or muscle tissue. It will take 48 to 72 hours for the patch to reach its full effectiveness. During that time, short-term analgesia such as morphine should be taken. Pain control and side effects should be monitored during the first days of medication changeover. Normally the patch should be changed every 72 hours; however, it can be changed every 48 hours if the patient is consistently having increased pain on the third day. Choose a different site for placement with each new application. If the skin becomes irritated, a steroid may be sprayed on the area. Let it dry before placing the new patch. All unused patches should also be destroyed when they are no longer needed. Additional medication can be provided for breakthrough pain. Wash your hands after handling the patches.

Necessary education for caregivers of hospice or palliative care patients

The caregiver of the hospice or palliative care patient needs specific education in a number of areas:
- Stress: The caregiver should be aware of the indications and effects of stress on the individual, patient, and family members, methods of dealing with stress, and when to ask for help.
- Community resources: Needs may be many and varied and the caregiver often needs assistance from outside agencies.
- Patient care: The caregiver should understand basic patient care, such as assisting the patient with bathing, dressing, transferring, and taking/administering medications. The

caregiver should also receive education regarding appropriate diet and nutrition, wound care, and any other necessary medical care (such as catheter care).

- Disease: The caregiver needs to be educated about the patient's disease and expected progression, as well as any complications that may occur.
- Death process: The caregiver must understand the signs of impending death and should learn what to expect in terms of both physical and mental changes.

Life completion and closure

The following are the developmental landmarks associated with life completion and closure:
- A sense of completion in all affairs, including worldly, community, and interpersonal relationships with family and friends. The individual must feel that they have taken care of all unfinished business.
- They feel a satisfaction in life and work. After reflecting on their lives, patients can accept themselves and their accomplishments as fulfilling and worthwhile.
- They can experience feelings of love and acceptance for self and others: pursuing worthiness, forgiveness, gratitude, closure, and resolution of past hurts and wrongs to bring about peace and satisfaction.
- The patient is able to identify a general understanding of the meaning and finality of life.
- They express a willingness to move forward into the unknown, accepting death and saying goodbye.

Advocating for a change in level of care

Advocating for the palliative care patient to have a change in the level of care includes discussing care needs and options with the patient and family to ascertain their feelings and wishes. It also includes discussing changes in the patient's condition and the patient's wishes with the physician. For a patient on palliative care, the change in level of care may involve:
- Lesser form of care: This change is indicated because the patient is responding well to treatment, such as may occur following chemotherapy for cancer.
- Hospice care: If the patient's condition has deteriorated and death is expected within 6 months, then hospice care provides more benefits than palliative care. Patients and family are often unaware of hospice care benefits, so providing information can help with decision making. Hospice care is appropriate when no further curative treatment is available or when a patient opts to discontinue curative treatments in favor of comfort care.

Advanced care planning

Discussions and communication about patient preferences are beneficial for both the patient and family and friends. Being open about the patient's needs and expectations allows for increased clarity of care goals and can facilitate access to needed services. Among important decisions to be made is to identify the primary decision maker when the patient is unable to make decisions, have a clear understanding of the disease process and limitations of the physical condition, place financial affairs in order, identify treatment preferences in writing, and communicate openly with one's physician about these expectations. Most patients want to be able to make funeral plans, to have a sense of completion, and to have a general understanding of the timing of death. They are less like to express personal fears or appear vulnerable to families, physicians, and other caregivers. Other factors to discuss include relief of pain and other distressing symptoms, and decisions about specific medical treatments including life-sustaining therapies, artificial feeding and hydration, and palliative and hospice care.

Advanced directives

The American Nurses Association states, "The nurse has a responsibility to facilitate informed decision making, including but not limited to advance directives." Advanced directives can take the form of either a living will or durable power of attorney. Advance directives are completed by the able and knowledgeable patient in order to guide the care of all other decision makers when the patient can no longer make decisions for himself. These end-of-life care options and the identified health care proxy listed in the advance directives can be revised by the patient if and when desired. Advance directives do not require authentication by an attorney.

Discussing DNR order with patient and family

In discussing a Do Not Resuscitate (DNR) order, Dr. Charles von Gunten recommended the steps:
1. Establish an appropriate setting where the patient feels comfortable.
2. Establish what the patient and family understand of the patient's condition. Build on current knowledge.
3. Find out what the patient's future expectations are.
4. Discuss the DNR order in a manner that the patient can understand given their present condition and expectations for the future. Use language that the patient can understand. Identify specific examples and options.
5. Discuss the parameters in which resuscitation would be considered.
6. Respond appropriately to the patient's emotions, and assist in developing a plan. Encourage and respect any responses. Clearly document the patient's wishes in the care plan.

Patient autonomy regarding life support

Autonomy is the basic right of an individual to choose freely. Patient autonomy means that the individual is able to make informed, voluntary decisions regarding his or her care based on personal convictions. In the presence of an ethical dilemma, such as withholding or withdrawing life support, there is a controversy between patient and physician autonomy, or professional and institutional integrity. Each individual in a given situation has his or her own ethical and cultural beliefs. Even though respect for patient autonomy is important, the health care worker cannot be obligated to perform treatments that he or she considers outside of their basic morals. While autonomy assumes a patient's innate right to make decisions for himself or herself, others may argue that no human being is entitled to determine matters of life and death.

Medical futility

Medical futility has many proposed definitions. In many cases, the definition is determined by the situation. When values are in conflict, questions of futility are often raised. Futility represents the acknowledgement that a particular therapy will not offer a benefit to the patient. With this acknowledgement it is determined that the treatment should not be provided. Parameters for this determination are wide. Some define futility as a success rate of less than 1% for a given treatment, or more broadly, therapy that it is outside of the community standards or the patient's goals for treatment. Often judgments of futility are based on the worth of possible goals weighed against known negative outcomes or potential for harm.

Addressing ethical issues in palliative care

Nurses can help address ethical issues by working closely with patients, families, and physicians within his or her scope of education, experience, and practice. The greatest nursing role during ethical dilemmas is providing patient and family education. This enables patients to consider all options and choose from those that fit within their value system, beliefs, and anticipated outcomes for their care. Nurses can provide unbiased, scientifically based information about all available options to be considered. Physicians are charged with determining the patient's competence and ability to make decisions for himself and establishing other means of decision making when necessary. Ethics consultations may be requested when difficult conflicts exist or dilemmas become complex with no clear answers.

Double effect

If a specific act has more than one potential effect, it can be considered ethical under the terms of double effect. To be qualified as a double effect, four basic conditions should be met.
- The nature of the act is morally good. The intentions of the act cannot have grounds in anything that is considered strictly prohibited or fundamentally wrong.
- The intent is good. There can be a potential for negative effects, but the core intent of the act is intended to be morally beneficial.
- Good can be obtained without the use of dire means. The intended relief of suffering cannot be achieved through unethical or harmful means.
- The balance of good is greater than the anticipated negative effects. This is sometimes referred to as the rule of proportionality.

A fifth condition is sometimes considered in that there are no other options available to obtain the needed good effect.

Patient Care: Life-Limiting Conditions in Adult Patients

Physical symptoms experienced by people who are actively dying

Imminent death is defined by physical signs and symptoms that indicate the anticipation of death within hours or days. The patient shows signs of profound weakness, requiring complete care. They appear gaunt and pale, have cool extremities, and lack interest in food or drink, with difficulty swallowing and significant decreases in intake. Changes in breathing patterns are also common, including dyspnea changing to an easier, shallow respiration with decreased oxygen concentration, and gurgling or gravely sounds in the back of the throat from excess secretions. There may be a transient improvement in comfort, pain experiences, and mental status, but the overall state is one varying in agitation, restlessness, delirium and confusion, increased pain, profound sleepiness with a reduction in awareness, difficulty concentrating, and disorientation to time and place. A semicomatose or fully comatose state may become present. The patient may also experience incontinence, and third-space fluids may be reabsorbed, decreasing the amount of swelling present. Pupils become fixed and dilated.

Death rattle

The death rattle is a term used to describe the gurgling or rattling noise made from the accumulation of excessive secretions in the throat. It is generally associated with the last stages of the dying process. During this time, the patient may lack the ability to swallow their secretions, causing the buildup of fluid. Other types of swallowing difficulties can produce this same effect. It is sometimes interpreted as the sound of choking and misidentified as the cause of death. Anticholinergic agents have antisecretory properties and should be given at the first sign of moisture. They can stop further fluid buildup but cannot dry up secretions already present. Fluids present in the mouth may be removed with suction or oral care. Agents that can be used include scopolamine, hyoscine hydrobromide, and atropine.

End stage disease progression of neurologic disorders

End-stage disease progression of neurologic disorders varies but there are some commonalities:
- Progressive weakness/disability: Ambulatory patients may progress to wheelchair bound or bedridden. Patients may be unable to manage personal care or any ADLs, such as eating, toileting, and bathing, without assistance. While range-of-motion and other exercises may help, the changes are usually not reversible, so the caregiver may need assistance to provide care.
- Speech impairment: The patient's speech may be difficult to understand or the patient may lose the ability to communicate verbally. Assistive devices, such as computerized systems, may help and the patient may be able to communicate through picture or letter boards.
- Dysphagia: The patient may choke easily and eventually lose the ability to swallow. Initially, the dysphagia may be controlled through changes in diet (soft or pureed foods) but eventually the patient may need a feeding tube to maintain nutrition and hydration.
- Respiratory distress: Positioning and oxygen administration may relieve respiratory distress, but those with severe impairment may require intubation and ventilation.

End-stage disease progression of cardiac disorders

End-stage disease progression of cardiac disorders often includes the following:
- Dyspnea: Opioids often help to relieve dyspnea. Other interventions include positioning the patient with head of bed elevated, using a fan aimed toward the patient's face, administering oxygen, and avoiding NSAIDS (which may reduce the effects of diuretics and other drugs). If dyspnea is related to pulmonary edema, diuretics and vasodilators may provide relief.
- Pain: This may be cardiac or edema-related, affecting the chest or the entire body. Opioids are generally the drugs of choice to relieve pain related to end-stage disease.
- Fatigue/Depression: Relieving other symptoms and providing both physical and emotional support may help to reduce fatigue and depression.
- Fluid retention: Elevating the legs to improve circulation and administration of diuretics and vasodilators (as for dyspnea) may provide some relief.
- General weakness: Patients will become bedbound as the condition progresses and unable to attend to ADLs without assistance.

End stage disease progression of oncologic disorders

End-stage disease oncologic disorders may vary depending on the type of cancer and the areas of metastasis but often includes the following:
- Pain: This is the most common complication and may be localized or generalized. Opioids are the treatment of choice, usually on a continuous round-the-clock schedule with additional doses for breakthrough pain at end-stage to provide as much comfort as possible.
- Nausea/Vomiting: Anti-emetics and/or medical marijuana may help to reduce nausea and vomiting. The patient's diet should be altered to include those foods the patient can best tolerate, often soft, bland or liquid foods.
- Dyspnea: Dyspnea is common, and supplementary oxygen may help to provide some relief.
- Confusion: Supportive care and reorienting the patient may help to reduce confusion, but confusion often persists, especially with high doses of opioids.
- Bowel/bladder dysfunction: This is common because of dehydration and opioid use. Stool softeners, laxatives and encouraging fluid intake may help. If the patient is still able to eat, adding yogurt, fiber, and prune juice to the diet may be helpful.

Leukemia

Leukemia is classified as acute or chronic depending on the type of cell that it originates from and the genetic chromosomal or growth factor deviation present in the malignant cells. Hematological malignancies evolve from immature blood cells, multiplying profusely and compromising the integrity of the normal blood cells. Clinical findings may include infection, anemia, fever, an enlarged liver, spleen, and kidneys, accompanied by pain or tenderness over the sternum or other bones and joints. The patient may complain of fatigue, lethargy, and unexplained bleeding and bruising. Further examination may reveal pallor, petechia, purpura, and bleeding mucous membranes. As normal blood cells become depleted, anemia, infection, and hemorrhage become more common and can result in death.

Lymphoma

Lymphoma can present as Hodgkin disease or non-Hodgkin lymphoma. Signs and symptoms of Hodgkin disease consist of painless lymph node swelling (though lymph nodes may become painful after alcohol consumption), generally in the upper body, general fatigue, rapid and unexplained weight loss, intermittent fevers, significant night sweats, frequent infections, itching without an apparent rash or other cause, and occasionally unexplained back pain. Occasional other complaints include upset stomach and bowel changes. Physical assessment may also reveal an enlarged liver or spleen. Night sweats and itching are less common with non-Hodgkin lymphoma. Other signs and symptoms remain the same. In later stages, anemia and thrombocytopenia may be present with either form of lymphoma.

Neurological symptoms of cerebral metastases

Brain metastasis occurs in up to 40% of all cancer patients. The neurological changes may be the first identified symptoms in some silent forms of cancer. Symptoms include headaches, nausea, vomiting, confusion, and lethargy. Headache is the initial complaint in approximately half of all patients. These are caused by an increased intracranial pressure from tumor growth, brain swelling, or a blockage on the cerebral spinal fluid pathway (hydrocephalus). The tumor can cause location-specific brain function disruptions, such as weakness, numbness, language deficits, visual disturbances, and other stroke-like symptoms. It can also lead to seizures in approximately 15% of affected patients. Behavior changes can include depression, apathy, memory problems, or changes in personality.

ALS

Amyotrophic lateral sclerosis (ALS) is a rapidly progressing degenerative neuromuscular disease with an unknown origin. The main area of involvement is the motor neurons of the brain and spinal cord. Approximately half of those patients presenting with ALS will have difficulty swallowing as their first symptom. Other patients will experience distal weakness. As the disease progresses, weakness affects both the upper and lower neurons. Death generally results from respiratory failure due to weakness in the diaphragm along with decreased laryngeal and lingual functionality. Swallowing and oral nourishment are of high concern for these patients. Loss of motility in the tongue and hypopharynx result in the loss of ability to manipulate food as well as creating speech and communication barriers.

Parkinson disease

Parkinson disease is a fairly common disease of the central nervous system. There is a slow progression of motor skill complications, including resting tremors, excessive slowness in activity, and rigidity. Classic signs include pill-rolling movements in the hands, loss of facial expression, difficulty initiating movements, and gait changes. Because of its slow progression, patients may initially present with generalized weakness, aching, fatigue, and malaise. A slight tremor of an extremity may also be noted. Symptoms result from an imbalance between dopamine-activated and acetylcholine-activated neural pathways in the basal ganglia and are generally found in people older than 65 years. Parkinson-like symptoms can also be caused by medication toxicity, head trauma, or other degenerative conditions.

Advanced renal cancer

Renal cancers generally occur asymptomatically in the early stages. Symptoms begin to appear as the condition worsens. Gross hematuria, dull, aching pain, and palpable abdominal mass are generally the first signs. When all three of these are evidenced in the patient, it is generally a well-advanced cancer. Hematuria is the most common symptom but may not be noticed until it has reached the gross stage where it is visible to the naked eye. Other late signs and symptoms can include fever, anemia, weight loss, night sweats, elevated erythrocyte sedimentation rate, dyspnea, hypertension, hypercalcemia, and polycythemia. Polycythemia may cause headaches, dizziness, vein inflammation, itchiness, and a general feeling of bloating. Hypercalcemia causes tiredness, decreased appetite, frequent urination, thirst, nausea, vomiting, confusion, difficulty concentrating, and constipation.

End stage liver failure symptoms

Fatigue, ascites (the collection of fluid in the abdominal cavity), and jaundice are the hallmark symptoms of end-stage liver failure. These symptoms generally result from a low or nonfunctioning lymphatic system. Other complications include patient complaints of itching, dark-colored urine, gray- or clay-colored stool, and easy bruising. As the disease further progresses, internal bleeding and mental confusion (encephalopathy) can develop, eventually leading to a hepatic coma. Sudden fever over 101°F, dyspnea, evident or suspected internal bleeding, severe abdominal pain, and severe dehydration are considered urgent conditions requiring additional medical treatment. Palliative care for many symptoms is available; in general, those with end-stage liver disease or failure would require a liver transplant in order to survive.

Effects of AIDS virus on patient's cells

The AIDS virus attaches itself to the CD4 cell surface protein of T-4 lymphocytes with a viral envelope of glycoprotein (gp120). This protein binds to CD4 receptors and coreceptors (CXCR4 and CCR5). HIV is a retrovirus that quickly infects circulating immune cells or finds safe harbors in body reservoirs that are inaccessible to drug therapy. The retrovirus uses an enzyme called reverse transcriptase to convert the HIV viral RNA to a viral DNA. This conversion allows the viral DNA to take over the host cell DNA of lymphocytes, macrophages, and other immune system cells. When the viral DNA has taken over, it produces viral proteins that assemble into virions using viral enzyme protease. Each reproductive cycle of HIV can produce up to 100 billion virions with minor protective mutations. The CD4 count indicates disease severity. A count of less than 500 cells/mm^3 is found in the early symptomatic stage. A count less than 200 cells/mm^3 and a viral load greater than 100,000/mL are found in the late symptomatic stage.

Infections and malignancies associated with AIDS

The AIDS patient is highly susceptible to many bacterial, viral, fungal, and parasitic infections as well as certain types of cancers, such as Kaposi sarcoma and CNS and non-Hodgkin lymphoma.
- Bacterial infections include Streptococcus pneumoniae, Mycobacterium avium-intracellulare (MAI) and Mycobacterium avium complex (MAC), tuberculosis (TB), salmonellosis, syphilis, and Bacillary angiomatosis.
- Viral infections include cytomegalovirus (CMV), viral hepatitis, herpes simplex virus (HSV), human papillomavirus (HPV), and progressive multifocal leukoencephalopathy (PML).

- Fungal infections include Candida albicans, Histoplasma capsulatum, and cryptococcal meningitis.
- Parasitic infections include Pneumocystis carinii pneumonia (PCP), toxoplasmosis, and cryptosporidium.

The rates of infection with these types of infections in AIDS patients far exceed the rates found within the general population.

AIDS dementia complex

The exact cause of AIDS dementia is unknown, but it is a primary result of the disease process itself. Current theories suggest that the HIV infection stimulates an invasion of macrophages in the brain (microglia). These release cytokines that directly damage the nervous tissue by disrupting the neurotransmitter functions and cause encephalopathy. This condition affects as many as 15% of all AIDS patients. Prognosis is poor and the disease is not reversible. However, retrovirals can delay its onset. Central nervous system HIV infection in children tends to have a more dramatic and pronounced effect than that in adults. AIDS dementia is characterized by gradual memory loss, decreased concentration, and cognition and mood disorders. The patient may also experience physical symptoms of ataxia, incontinence, and seizures.

Palliative sedation

Palliative sedation is a treatment method focused on controlling and easing symptoms that have proven otherwise refractory or unendurable in nature. This process was originally named terminal sedation. It was changed to palliative sedation to emphasize the differences between symptom management and euthanasia. The purpose of palliative sedation is symptom control; it does not hasten or cause death. Through the monitored use of medications such as midazolam or propofol, relief can be provided through varying levels of unconsciousness. Among terminally ill patients, palliative sedation is most often used to calm persistent agitation and restlessness. The second most frequent need is for pain control, followed by confusion, shortness of breath, muscle twitching or seizures, and anguish.

Terminal weaning and terminal extubation

Terminal weaning represents the slow withdrawal of life-supporting ventilators. This is normally performed by gradually reducing the amount of inspired oxygen (FIO_2) and/ or the programmed ventilator rate. This process leads to the eventual development of hypoxemia and hypercarbia that is fatal to the patient. This reduction of mechanical ventilator settings occurs gradually over the course of many hours. Terminal extubation, in contrast, is the abrupt withdrawal of the endotracheal tube and subsequently the mechanical ventilator support. This removal of assistance, which the patient is dependent on for life, causes death. This process is generally initiated after administration of sedative and/or analgesics to the patient. Both processes are subject to ethical question and debate. Therefore, practices will vary between individual practitioners and organizations.

Patient Care: Pain Management

Visceral pain

Visceral pain is associated with the internal organs. It can be very different depending on the affected organ. Not all internal organs are sensitive to pain (some lack nociceptors, such as the spleen, kidney, and pancreas), and may withstand a great deal of damage without causing pain. Other internal organs, such as the stomach, bladder, and ureters, can create significant pain from even the slightest damage. Visceral pain generally has a poorly defined area. It is also capable of referring pain to other remote locations away from the area of injury. It is described as a squeezing or cramping, a deep ache within the internal organs. The patient may complain of a generalized "sick" feeling or have nausea and vomiting. Visceral pain generally responds well to treatment with opioids.

Neuropathic pain

Neuropathic pain results from injury to the nervous system. This can result from cancer cells compressing the nerves or spinal cord, from actual cancerous invasion into the nerves or spinal cord, or from chemical damage to the nerves caused by chemotherapy and radiation. Other causes include diabetes- and alcohol-related damage, trauma, neuralgias, or other illnesses affecting the neural path either centrally or peripherally. When the nerves become damaged, they are unable to carry accurate information. This results in more severe, distinct pain messages. The nerves may also relay pain messages long after the original cause of the pain is resolved. It can be described as sharp, burning, shooting, shocking, tingling, or electrical in nature. It may travel the length of the nerve path from the spine to a distal body part such as a hand, or down the buttocks to a foot. NSAIDs and opioids are generally ineffective against neuropathic pain, though adjuvants may enhance the therapeutic effect of opioids. Nerve blocks may also be used.

Somatic pain

Somatic pain refers to messages from pain receptors located in the cutaneous or musculoskeletal tissues. When the pain occurs within the musculoskeletal tissue, it is referred to as deep somatic pain. Metastasizing cancers commonly cause deep somatic pain. Surface pain refers to pain concentrated in the dermis and cutaneous layers such as that caused by a surgical incision. Deep somatic pain is generally described as a dull, throbbing ache that is well focused on the area of trauma. It responds well to opioids. Surface somatic pain is also directly focused on the injury. It is frequently described as sharper than deep somatic pain. It may also present as a burning or pricking sensation.

Nociceptive pain

Nociceptive pain is an umbrella term for pain caused by stimulation of the neuroreceptor. This stimulation is a direct result of tissue injury and follows four stages: transduction where a change occurs, transmission where the impulse is transferred along the neural path, modulation or translation of the signal, and perception by the patient. The severity of pain is proportionate to the extent of the injury. Nociceptive pain can be subdivided into two classifications: somatic and visceral pain. Somatic pain is located in the cutaneous tissues, bone joints, and muscle tissues.

Visceral pain is specific to internal organs protected by a layer of viscera such as the cardiovascular, respiratory, gastrointestinal, or genitourinary systems. Both types are treatable with opioids.

Nociceptors

Nociceptors are the primary neurons, or sensory receptors, responding to stimulus in the skin, muscle, and joints, as well as the stomach, bladder, and uterus. These neurons have specialized responses for mechanical, thermal, or chemical stimuli. The neuron stimulation is a direct result of tissue injury and follows four stages: transduction where a change occurs, transmission where the impulse is transferred along the neural path, modulation or translation of the signal, and perception by the patient. When injury occurs, the nociceptors initiate the process that begins depolarization of the peripheral nerve. Nociceptors may consist of either A axons or C axons. The message passes along the neural pathway and creates a perception of pain. A axons carry these pain messages at a much faster rate than C axons.

Physical indications of pain

The best assessment of the patient's pain is his own report. All other information is assessed as supporting this report. However, when this is method is restricted or unavailable, physical signs and symptoms can help the nurse's assessment capabilities. It is important to be familiar with the patient's baseline or resting information to give a clear picture of the changes the body may go through when experiencing significant pain. Systolic blood pressure, heart rate and respirations may all increase above the patient's normal parameters. Tightness or tension may be felt in major muscle groups. Posturing can also occur: the patient may guard areas of the body, curl around themselves in a "fetal" position or hold only certain body portions rigid. Calling out, increased volume in speech and moaning can also be indicators. Facial expressions such as flat affect or grimacing and distraction from their surroundings also indicate a significant increase in stressful stimulus.

Areas to address when assessing pain

Information concerning a patient's pain can be gathered from a variety of sources including observations, interviews with the patient and family, medical records and observations of other health care providers. However, it is important to remember that each patient's pain is subjective and personal. Pain is defined as whatever the patient says it is. Having the patient give parameters of location, duration or length of the pain, onset or when it began, and intensity as defined by pain assessment scales can all be beneficial in forming a treatment plan based on the patients needs. Pain is also influenced by psychological, social, and spiritual factors. Behavioral, psychological and subjective assessment information such as physical demeanor and vital signs can be helpful in further defining a patient's pain parameters.

Importance of pain assessments in non-verbal patients

As many as 90% of all advanced disease patients will experience some level of pain. The hospice and palliative care philosophy focuses on the relief of pain and provision for comfort measures for all patients who desire it to improve quality of life. Each patient has the right to accept or refuse treatment for their pain. This becomes difficult when the patient is unable to communicate their desires and pain level. It can be assumed that if a patient was experiencing pain when able to communicate, they will continue to experience pain when the ability to communicate has be compromised- pain will be present even in an unconscious state. Changes from previous behavioral, psychological and subjective and objective assessment data provide the supporting information for continued pain assessments in the non-verbal patient.

Unidimensional tools for pain assessment

The following are three unidimensional tools for pain assessment:
- Numeric rating scale (NRS): The NRS is the most widely known rating scale. Patients are asked to rate their pain on a 0 to 10 scale or 0 to 5 scale. Zero is for no pain and the highest number is the worst pain possible.
- Visual analog scale (VAS): The VAS is a 10 cm line, marked on one end for no pain and the other end for most severe pain. The patient indicates the place on the line where he feels his pain is represented. The line is then measured to the indicated point and assigned a score.
- Categorical scales: Categorical scales allow patients to rate pain intensity with either verbal or visual responses. The verbal scale introduced by Melzack and Torgerson uses five verbal descriptors (mild, discomforting, distressing, horrible, and excruciating). The Faces Pain Scale (FPS) and the Wong-Baker Faces Rating Scale use both words and corresponding images of various facial expressions (eg, frowning, grimacing, smiling) for the patients to choose from.

Core principles of pain assessment and management as defined by the Joint Commission

All patients have the right to appropriate assessment and management of pain. Caregivers should encourage all patients to report their pain and follow through with pain-relieving treatments. Assessments for pain must be appropriate for the individual patient and address all aspects of their pain. Both the patient and family should be included in the assessment process. The most accurate indicator of pain is the patient's own description. It is always subjective; the clinician should accept and respect the patient's report of pain. Each person's pain experience is unique and dependent on many contributing factors such as heredity, energy level, coping skills, and prior experiences. Physiological and behavioral observations should not replace information obtained directly from the patient when it can be communicated. Pain can be present without physiological evidence or cause. Pain in such cases should not be immediately assigned to a psychological cause. Chronic pain can create an overall lower threshold of tolerance for pain and other stimuli. Unrelieved pain has adverse effects on all aspects of the patient's life.

ABCDE mnemonic approach to pain assessment

As a reflection on the national trend toward higher quality pain control within the health care setting, The Agency for Healthcare Research and Quality (AHRQ) recommends the following mnemonic for assessing and managing pain.
- A. Ask regularly and consistently. Use the same systematic approach every time pain is assessed.
- B. Believe the patient's report of pain and how it is best relieved.
- C. Choose appropriate pain control options according to the needs of the patient, family, and setting.
- D. Deliver pain relief in a timely, consistent, and coordinated manner.
- E. Empower the patient and family with information and an active voice in their care plan. As much as possible, care and pain relief should always be patient driven.

Multidimensional tools for pain assessment

The following are multidimensional tools used to assess pain:
- Initial Pain Assessment Tool: This tool is specific to the initial patient evaluation. It assesses the characteristics of the pain, the patient's manner of expressing pain, and the effects of the pain of the patient's quality of life. A diagram is used to indicate pain locations and a scale rates pain intensity. It also provides for additional observations, comments and plans.
- Brief Pain Inventory (BPI): This tool is meant to quickly identify both pain intensity and its related restrictions. It consists of a series of questions about the patient's pain over the last 24 hours including location, intensity, quality of life, type and patient response to any treatments.
- McGill Pain Questionnaire (MPQ): The MPQ tool assesses pain on three levels: sensory, affective, and evaluative. It consists of identifying words selected by the patient to describe their pain and can be used in combined with other tools. The MPQ is available in both long and short forms.

Assessment tools to use with cognitively impaired or nonverbal patients

The following are types of assessment tools available for use with cognitively impaired or nonverbal patients:
- Discomfort Scale for Dementia of the Alzheimer Type (DS-DAT): For use with elderly persons experiencing dementia, decreased cognition, and decreased verbalization.
- Assessment of Discomfort in Dementia Protocol (ADD): Particularly designed for use with patients exhibiting difficult behaviors.
- Checklist of Nonverbal Pain Indicators (CNPI): Pain measurement with cognitive impairment
- Noncommunicative Patient's Pain Assessment Instrument (NOPPAIN): Specifically for use by nursing assistants.
- Pain Assessment for the Dementing Elderly (PADE): Assessing physical pain behaviors
- Pain Assessment Tool in Confused Older Adults (PATCOA): Focuses on the observation of nonverbal cues.
- Pain Assessment in Advanced Dementia (PAINAD): Adapted from the DS-DAT
- Pain Assessment Checklist for Seniors with Limited Ability to Communicate (PACSLAC): To assess common and subtle symptoms.
- Abbey Pain Scale: For late-stage dementia in nursing home environments.

Neuropathic Pain Scale

The Neuropathic Pain Scale was recently developed in response to the need for a way to assess and provide information about the specific types and degrees of sensations experienced by patients living with neuropathic pain. Its goal is to evaluate 8 common qualities of neuropathic pain. These sensations are sharp, dull, hot, cold, sensitive, itchy, deep, and surface. The patient is asked to rate each sensation on a number scale from 0 to 10. Zero represents none, 10 is the worst imaginable sensation. Though still early in its therapeutic availability and uses, studies suggest that this form is easy to use and sensitive to the specific and diagnostic pain needs of the neuropathic pain patient.

Assessing pain in pediatric patients

When assessing the pediatric patient, the nurse must take into consideration the chronological and developmental age of the child. These help determine which measure the child might use to express pain, as well as treatments that might prove most successful. Assessment parameters must also include the presence of and parameters surrounding chronic illness, as well as neurological impairment. Identify the underlying cause of the pain, what nonpharmacological measures have been tried for pain control, and what methods can be used to deliver pharmacological interventions. The weight of the child in kilograms determines the appropriate dosages of medications. If the child is able to speak, do the child and the parents speak the same language as the health care provider, and are there any other obvious barriers to communication or pain relief measures?

QUESTT pediatric pain assessment tool

QUESTT is designed to focus on assessment, action, and consequent reassessment for results.
- Q – Question both the child and parent about the pain experience.
- U – Use assessment tools and rating scales that are appropriate to the developmental stage and situation and understanding of the child.
- E – Evaluate the patient for both behavioral and physiological changes.
- S – Secure the parent's participation in all stages of the pain evaluation and treatment process.
- T – Take the cause of the pain into consideration during the evaluation and choice of treatment methods.
- T – Take action to treat the pain appropriately, and then evaluate the results on a regular basis.

Health care professional and system barriers to optimal pain assessments

On the nursing assessment level, multiple factors contribute to variances and substandard pain assessments. Some nurses fail to recognize the importance of a full pain assessment. This may be the result of inadequate knowledge, or a perceived lack of time necessary to conduct a pain assessment. It is therefore given a low priority in the nursing care plan. Other interpersonal factors may also interfere. The nurse may have an inability to establish rapport or empathize with the patient. Personal prejudice and bias when dealing with certain patients may also interfere with overall care. The healthcare system can also fail to place a level of importance on full pain assessments by a lack of provider accountability, policies, criteria or availability of pain assessment tools.

Patient, family and societal barriers to optimal pain assessments

Because of the highly subjective and personal nature of pain, the patient may inadvertently sabotage attempts at a full pain assessment and subsequent treatment. If there is a lack of rapport with the health care staff, the patient may be unwilling to communicate the extent of his pain, or fear that he will be seen as a "bother" or drug seeker. The patient's overall attitude may be depressed and fatalistic, causing him to feel that the pain is inevitable and must be tolerated, or he may feel that treatments will be ineffective. He may also lack understanding about effective treatment methods. Cultural, religious, and age-related factors create additional barriers. The patient may lack effective communication skills necessary to relate what he is feeling or have unfounded beliefs about pain and its treatment.

Sources of pain HIV/AIDS patient

Sources of pain that may be present for the HIV/AIDS patient:
- Aphthous ulcer and oral candidiasis produce painful sores within the oral cavity; dysphagia may also be experienced.
- Arthralgia is joint pain with heat, redness, tenderness, loss of motion, and swelling. Cryptococcal meningitis is a life-threatening fungal infection resulting in headache, dizziness, and stiff neck. Coma and death can occur.
- Hepatotoxicity is liver damage resulting in nausea, vomiting, abdominal pain, loss of appetite, diarrhea, fatigue and weakness, jaundice, swelling, and weight gain.
- Herpes simplex virus 2 (HSV-2) produces painful sores around the anus or genitals.
- Isosporiasis is a gastrointestinal infection. Diarrhea, fever, headache, abdominal pain, vomiting, and weight loss result.
- Myalgia is the condition of muscle pain and tenderness, general discomfort, and weakness throughout entire body.
- Neuralgia and peripheral neuropathy are sources of chronic nerve pain.
- Stevens-Johnson syndrome (SJS) is a reaction to medications and creates a severe to fatal skin rash with red, blistered, and painful spots on skin, mouth, eyes, genital, and moist areas of the body, or internal organs.

Factors influencing perception of pain

In conjunction with the goal of holistic care in the hospice and palliative care settings, it is important to assess and treat all aspects of the patient's pain. Unrelieved pain has adverse effects on all aspects of the patient's life. Pain does not occur in isolation. Its intensity is an individual perception based on physical, psychological, social, and spiritual factors. Pain can be present without a known or visible cause. The patient's total pain response is based on many contributing factors, such as heredity, energy level, coping skills, support systems, and prior experiences, as well as tissue damage and other physical influences. Other symptoms and concerns experienced by the patient compound the suffering associated with pain. Chronic pain can create an overall lower threshold of tolerance for pain and other stimuli.

Influence of gender on pain experience

Gender can affect pain sensitivity, tolerance, distress, and exaggeration of pain, and the patient's willingness to report pain, as well as displayed nonverbal cues concerning the pain experience. Studies indicate that women generally have lower pain thresholds and less tolerance for noxious stimuli or pain factors that hinder them from doing things they enjoy. Women seek help for pain-related problems sooner than men and respond better to therapy. Women also experience more visceral pain than men. Men are more prone to experience somatic pain and show more stoicism regarding pain experiences than women. Neuropathic pain seems to be experienced equally between men and women. Nurses need to be careful that biases concerning gender experiences with pain do not skew their assessments of pain. However, they need to be aware that pain experiences are always individual and may differ between the sexes.

Cultural considerations for pain management

American Indian and Alaskan natives are unwilling to show pain or request medications. Pain is a difficulty that must be endured rather than treated.

Asian and Pacific Islanders do not vocalize pain and may have an interest in pursuing nontraditional and nonpharmacological treatments, such as acupuncture, to help relieve pain.

Black and African American cultures tend to openly express their pain but still believe that it is to be endured. They may avoid medication because of personal fears of addition or cultural stigmatism.

Hispanic cultures value the ability to endure pain and suffering as a personal quality of strength. Expression of pain, especially for a male, is considered a sign of weakness. They may feel that pain is a form of godly punishment or trial.

Medications useful in treating neuropathic pain

Treatment options for neuropathic pain are often different from the methods used to treat other types of pain. The three drug classes most commonly used and proven effective for treating neuropathic pain are anticonvulsants, anesthetics, and antidepressants. Some are given on an as-needed basis but most require consistent dosing with 24-hour symptom control. Examples of the most common medications include amitriptyline, nortriptyline, duloxetine, gabapentin, topical lidocaine, opioids, and pregabalin. Medication choice is dependent on factors such as the type and progression of the disorder and the associated physical and emotional problems, such as nerve injury, muscle weakness, or spasms, anxiety, depression, or sleep disturbances.

Guidelines for opioid use

Opioid analgesic therapy is a widely used method of chronic pain control. By adhering to clinical guidelines, pain control can be safely optimized. Intramuscular administration should be used as a last resort except in the presence of a "pain emergency" when no other treatment is readily available. Such cases are rare since subcutaneous delivery is almost always an alternative. Noninvasive routes such as transdermal and transmucosal, which bypass the enteral route, are optimal for continuous pain control and are often effective in eliminating breakthrough pain as well. Changing from one opioid to another, or altering the delivery method, may become necessary under the assumption that incomplete cross-tolerance among opioids occurs. Changing analgesics or method of delivery may result in a decreased drug requirement. When altering opioid delivery regimens, use morphine equivalents as the common factor for all dose conversions. This method will help reduce medication errors. Side effects such as sedation, constipation, nausea, and myoclonus should be anticipated in every care plan, and require both prevention and treatment methods.

Opioid use during the last few hours of life

Assessment of pain continues in the last hours of life and medication is adjusted according to assessment. Pain does not necessarily increase as death approaches. It can be assumed that if pain was present prior to loss of consciousness it will continue in the patient's unconscious state. It should be assessed for and treated accordingly. Research has confirmed that administering opioids at the end of life does not hasten nor prolong the dying process. The patient's prior medication regimen should be continued. However, adjustments may be made in consideration of reduced renal or hepatic clearance. The route of administration should also be assessed for appropriateness and adjusted as needed (eg, loss of consciousness, inability to swallow).

Oral transmucosal fentanyl citrate

Oral transmucosal fentanyl citrate consists of fentanyl on an oral applicator. The patient applies the dosage (starting at 200 mcg) to the buccal mucosa between the cheek and gum for rapid absorption and subsequent pain relief. This makes transmucosal fentanyl particularly useful for managing breakthrough pain. Pain relief generally begins within 5 minutes; the patient should be instructed to wait 15 minutes after the previous dose has been completed before taking another dose. Swallowing even part of the dose rather than having it completely absorbed through the oral mucosa can affect the timing of pain relief onset. Peak effect occurs in 20 to 40 minutes with the total pain relief duration lasting 2 to 3 hours. Side effects can include somnolence, nausea, and dizziness. Consuming drinks such as coffee, tea, and juices that alter the oral secretion pH can also alter the absorption rate of transmucosal fentanyl.

Methadone

Methadone is useful for treating severe or chronic pain and may be particularly helpful in the presence of neuropathic pain. It has a long-acting pain relief factor for a lower cost than many comparable medications. However, the exact dosing ratios with morphine remain unclear within the available research. Metabolism of methadone can also be swayed (either increased or decreased) by many other medications normally taken by patients with chronic conditions. Methadone can be used to treat opioid addiction. US law for the prescription of methadone for addiction in detoxification or maintenance programs requires a special license and patient enrollment. The words "for pain" need to be clearly stated in the prescription. Methadone can cause drowsiness, weakness, headache, nausea, vomiting, constipation, sweating, and flushing, as well as sedation, decreased respirations, or an irregular heart rate.

Oxycodone

Oxycodone, a synthetic formulation, is a long-acting opioid for moderate to severe pain relief. Side effects are similar to those of morphine. It has a similar pain relief ratio, with the possibility of less nausea and vomiting. Because if its extended-release nature, the medication cannot be cut or crushed for administration. Oxycodone does not carry any greater addiction risk than other types of opioids; however, public sensationalism related to this formulation may create hesitation for use among patient. Pharmacies may also limit the amount of this medication they will make available to an individual. Oxycodone should be used cautiously in patients with a history of hypothyroidism, Addison disease, urethral stricture, prostatic hypertrophy, or lung or liver disease.

Hydromorphone

Hydromorphone is available as tablets, liquid, suppository, and parenteral formulations. It offers the advantage of being synthetic, allowing for its use in the presence of a true morphine allergy. It is also helpful when significant side effects have occurred in the past or pain has been inadequately controlled with other medications. It may also be useful for controlling cough. However, neurotoxicity may occur, particularly myoclonus, hyperalgesia, and seizures. It should also be used cautiously in the presence of kidney, liver, heart, and thyroid disease, seizures disorders, respiratory disease, prostatic hypertrophy, or urinary problems. Common side effects include dizziness, lightheadedness, and drowsiness, upset stomach if taken without food, vomiting, and constipation.

Breakthrough pain

The three basic types of breakthrough pain are discussed below:
- Incident Pain: Pain that can be specifically tied to an activity or event, such as a dressing change or physical therapy. These events can be anticipated and treated with a rapid-onset, short-acting analgesic just prior to the painful event.
- Spontaneous Pain: This type of pain is unpredictable and cannot be pinpointed to a relationship with any certain time or event. There is no way to anticipate spontaneous pain. In the presence of neuropathic pain, adjuvant therapy may be useful. Otherwise a rapid-onset, short-acting analgesic is used.
- End-of-Dose Failure: Pain that specifically occurs at the end of a routine analgesic dosing cycle when medication blood levels begin to taper off. Careful evaluation of end-of-dose failure can help prevent it sooner. It may indicate an increased dose tolerance and the need for medication dose alterations.

Prescribing controlled substances to patients with advanced illness and addiction challenges

In the presence of addiction challenges it become important to choose a long-acting opioid that can facilitate around the clock dosing and minimize the need for short-term medications used for "breakthrough" doses. Short-term medication use should be very limited or eliminated entirely if possible. Whenever possible nondrug adjuvants such as relaxation techniques, distraction, biofeedback, TNS, and therapeutic communication in place of short-term medications. When short-term medication therapy is needed, a nonopioid is best. Limit the amount of medication available to the patient at any given time and monitor for compliance with pill counts and urine toxicology screens as necessary. In some instances, a referral to an addictions specialist is recommended.

Morphine for chronic cancer pain

One advantage of morphine for chronic cancer pain is that it has no ceiling dose. As tolerance to the medication increases or the disease progresses in severity, the dose can be gradually increased to an infinite level. It is also available in many different forms for administration, including intravenous, intramuscular, immediate release, sustained release, long-acting, liquid oral preparations, and suppositories. Morphine is often used as the equivalency standard for other opioid analgesics. Common side effects of morphine include sedation, respiratory depression, itching, nausea, chronic spasms or twitching of muscle groups, and constipation. Constipation is experienced by all patients receiving opioids. This inevitability should be planned for and treated aggressively. Hallucinations are common when morphine is initiated. After the first few days, most patients will overcome the respiratory depression, nausea, itching, and extreme sedation.

Acetaminophen use

Acetaminophen (APAP) remains one of the safest analgesics for long-term use. It can be used to treat mild pain or as an adjuvant with other analgesics for more severe pain. Nonspecific musculoskeletal pain and osteoarthritis are particularly responsive to APAP therapy. Acetaminophen also has a limited anti-inflammatory nature.
Acetaminophen should, however, be used cautiously in persons with altered liver or kidney function, as well as those with a history of significant alcohol use, regardless of liver function compromise. It should be dosed separately from any opioid analgesic, which should be given separately as well. This allows for individual titration of each drug to assess the individual needs and side effects separately.

- 33 -

Ketamine

Ketamine treatment begins with an initial bolus of 0.1 mg/kg IV. If there is no improvement, a second bolus, with double the dosage, is provided in 5 minutes. This can be repeated as needed. Boluses should be followed by a decrease in the patient's current opioid dose by 50% and an infusion of ketamine. Infusion dosing for ketamine is 0.015 mg/kg/min, or about 1 mg/min for a 70 kg person. If IV access cannot be attained, subcutaneous infusion is a possibility with dosing of 0.3 to 0.5 mg/kg. Consider concurrent treatment with a benzodiazepine to prevent hallucinations or frightful dreams and observe for increased secretions. These secretions may be treated with glycopyrrolate, scopolamine, or atropine as needed.

Meperidine

The clinical practice guidelines from the American Pain Society strongly discourage the use of meperidine, especially in the long-term palliative care setting. Meperidine does not have a long-lasting analgesic effect; it only lasts for 2 to 3 hours. Repeated doses may also lead to central nervous system toxicity. This toxicity is the result of ineffective metabolite clearance. Individuals with renal insufficiency are unable to excrete the byproduct of meperidine from their system. The accumulation of this byproduct, normeperidine, in the body results in chronic muscle twitching or new-onset seizures. The metabolites of meperidine have also recently been linked with an increased pain perception and intensity. Normeperidine toxicity is not easily reversed and does not respond to naloxone.

Ketorolac

Ketorolac is an NSAID often used for its analgesic, antipyretic, and anti-inflammatory properties. It acts by inhibiting the synthesis of prostaglandins within the body. Though its therapeutic use is generally limited to short-term therapy of 5 days or less, it is the only NSAID available in oral, intramuscular, and ophthalmic solutions. The ophthalmic solution is effective in treating general eye pain as well as irritation related to seasonal allergies. Like most NSAIDs, it is used cautiously, or contraindicated in the patient with renal disease or dysfunction. The most common side effects include edema, hypertension, rash, nausea, constipation, diarrhea, vomiting, drowsiness, dizziness, and headache. The following serious risk factors are related to ketorolac: stomach ulcerations, bleeding, and perforation, renal damage, and hemorrhage.

NSAID use

Patients may benefit from NSAID use because of the anti-inflammatory, analgesic, and antipyretic properties. NSAIDs tend to be the first line of defense against pain caused by inflammatory conditions. They may also be used in conjunction with opioid therapy to reduce the amount of opioid needed. Adversely, gastrointestinal bleeding or ulceration, decreased renal function, and impaired platelet aggregation may occur. Studies have also indicated that the therapeutic affects of NSAIDs may not extend beyond six to twelve months of use. Short-term memory loss may occur in older patients. There may be an increased cardiovascular risk with prolonged use. Patients allergic to sulfa drugs can also experience a cross-sensitivity to some types of NSAIDs.

Dosages for morphine, codeine, hydromorphone, and levorphanol

The dosages for both the enteral and parenteral routes of morphine, codeine, hydromorphone, and levorphanol are compared below:
- Morphine: Enteral dosage is 30 mg (available as continuous and sustained-release formulations to last 12 to 24 hours); parenteral dosage is 10 mg.
- Codeine: Enteral dosage is 200 mg (not generally recommended); parenteral dosage is 130 mg.
- Hydromorphone: Enteral dosage is 7.5 mg (available as a continuous-release formula lasting 24 hours); parenteral dosage is 1.5 mg.
- Levorphanol: In acute pain episodes, enteral dosage is 4 mg; parenteral dosage is 2 mg. For chronic pain, dosage is equivalent for both enteral and parenteral at 1 mg. Levorphanol has a long half-life, increasing the chances of dosage accumulation over time.
- Adhering to the statement "If the gut works, use it," as much as 90 percent of all patients will at least start out able to use oral medications instead of other routes.

Calculation process for converting medication regimen between two opioids

Calculate the current 24-hour drug dose, or the total amount given in a 24-hour period. Multiply the current 24-hour dose times the ratio of the 24-hour equivalent dose for the new drug over the 24-hour equivalent of the old drug. This calculation provides the equivalent 24-hour dose for the new drug. Divide the new dose amount by the number of doses to be provided during the day. This amount equals the new target dosage.

$$current\ 24hr\ dose \times \frac{new\ drug\ 24hr\ equiv\ dose}{current\ drug\ 24\ hr\ equiv\ dose} = new\ 24hr\ dose$$

$$\frac{new\ 24hr\ dose}{doses\ per\ day} = new\ target\ dosage$$

Pain documentation in the medical record

Pain documentation in the medical record should include the following:
- An initial comprehensive pain assessment with the current pain management regimen and the patient's past experience with pain and its control.
- Patient goals and expectations for pain management should be addressed.
- Current analgesic routine and any concerns regarding drugs in use should be addressed.
- Bodily functions affected by medications are to be reviewed, including bowels, balance, and other quality of life issues.
- Interdisciplinary progress notes include recurrent pain assessments with baseline pain scores, breakthrough pain episodes, timing, severity, and related causes, and treatments.
- Any pain treatments, including nonpharmacological, timing, and results are documented.
- Related pain factors, such as sleep, activity levels, social interaction, and mood, are also important to note.
- Patient teaching interventions should be described and evaluated for effectiveness.
- Lastly, adverse effects, such as changes in bowel function, sedation, nausea, and vomiting, should be anticipated in the care plan, frequently assessed, and treated with accompanying documentation.

Measures taken when faced with pain crisis

Assess for a change in the mechanism or location of the pain, and attempt to differentiate between terminal anxiety or agitation and the physical causes of pain. Begin with a rapid increase in opioid treatment. If the pain is unresponsive to opioid titration, switching to benzodiazepines, such as diazepam and lorazepam, may produce a more effective response. If terminal symptoms remain unresponsive, assess for drug absorption. While invasive routes of medication delivery are generally avoided unless necessary, the only guaranteed route of drug delivery is the IV route. If there is any question about absorption, it is appropriate to establish parenteral access. IM delivery should be considered as a last resort. When all accessible resources have been exhausted, seek a pain management consultation as quickly as possible. Alternative methods of terminal pain control include radiotherapy, anesthetic, or neuroablative procedures.

Treatments for bone pain

Treatment options may depend on the causative agent related to the pain, such as the primary cancer site, severely weakened bones, or fractures. Systemic treatment choices include chemotherapy, radiation, and hormone therapy. Hormone therapy is used in the presence of estrogen and androgen receptors within the cancer cells. Bisphosphonates, such as ibandronate, zoledronate, and alendronate, may help strengthen the bones, slow damage, and prevent fractures; they can also help reduce pain. However, side effects can include fatigue, fever, nausea, vomiting, and anemia. Surgery may also be considered to remove cancerous cells or reinforce weakened areas of bone. Opioids and NSAIDs/COX-2 inhibitors are most often used for pain relief and need to be provided on a consistent basis.

Morphine combined with ibuprofen provides the benefit of a centrally acting opioid with a peripherally acting NSAID. Ibuprofen also acts as an effective adjuvant analgesic agent to enhance the relief provided by the opioid without increasing opioid side effects.

Quality pain management in palliative care setting

Individual patient needs, including cost, practicality, and convenience, should be taken into account with every prescription. Monitor the patient status frequently and adjust analgesics based on patient goals and the results of full pain assessments, including needs for supplemental analgesics, sleep, emotions, and quality-of-life factors. Around-the-clock pain relief should be provided in the form of sustained-release preparations and consistent dosing schedules. Immediate-release options should also be provided to accommodate for episodes of breakthrough pain. Avoid mixing agonist-antagonist opioids. Monitor for drug-drug and drug-disease interactions. Actively manage known side effects. Be familiar with the additional resources of pain management experts in your care community and make referrals as needed when pain cannot be adequately controlled using standard, reasonable guidelines and interventions.

Adjuvants

Adjuvant is defined as a complimentary treatment used in an effort to reduce and supplement current pharmacological responses. In immunology, chemicals such as aluminum hydroxide and aluminum phosphate are added to an antigen to cause a greater stimulation of the body's immunological responses by increasing the size of the antigen. This process makes it easier for the body's B lymphocytes and phagocytes to recognize antigen. This process is not effective with all antigens and cannot stimulate T-lymphocyte activity. In the area of pain control, adjuvants are generally used in conjunction with opioids to reduce the amount of medication required and enhance the overall analgesic effects. Pharmacological choices for increased pain control include antidepressants, anticonvulsants, and corticosteroids. Nonpharmacologic treatments can also be used as adjuvants, especially with pain control. The patient may gain better pain control with the addition of therapies, such as meditation, hot or cold application, or acupuncture.

Complementary and alternative medicine in palliative care

The patient may choose to explore complementary and alternative medicine for a variety of reasons. Given a poor prognosis, patients may attempt to focus on ways to improve their overall health, reduce side effects of medical treatments or the disease process, and improve the quality of their life. Approaches they feel are more in their control than medical treatments and interventions can help alleviate feelings of helplessness or hopelessness. It allows them to feel they are taking an active role in their care. Exploration of complementary and alternative medicine may also evolve from suggestions from friends or family; philosophical and cultural factors may also come into play. There is a desire to be sure that they have "tried everything," hoping to alter the course of disease progression. At times, there may be a mistrust or lack of faith in traditional medical treatments and a desire to treat the disease process in more "natural" ways. The patient may also feel that alternative medicine is less expensive and more accessible than traditional physicians and medical care.

Non-pharmacologic interventions appropriate for assisting in pain control

Multiple factors contribute to pain, so nondrug therapies such as cognitive-behavioral techniques and physical measures can serve as supplemental pain control measures, in turn reducing the amount of analgesics required by the patient. Cognitive-behavioral therapies are used to improve coping and relaxation techniques. These can include guided imagery, hypnosis, biofeedback, distraction with music or humor, prayer or other spiritual routines, simple exercises, rest, breathing exercises, and meditation. Even simple patient education about the nature and causes of pain can help patients feel more in control and less anxious in dealing with that pain. Physical measures include heat and cold, massage, reflexology, acupuncture, chiropractic, transcutaneous electrical nerve stimulation (TENS). In cases of refractory pain, nerve blocks and cordotomy may also be viable surgical options for pain management.

Concerns surrounding use of pain medications with end-of-life patients

Research has proven that controlling pain with medication does not shorten or extend the life span. Judicious use of pain medication cannot hasten the patient's death. Opioids are the most common medications used for severe pain in hospice or palliative care settings. Methadone is a common opioid choice since it is safe when used appropriately and inexpensive. Addiction and adverse effects are other frequent concerns raised by patients and family. These can also be positively addressed. Addiction to opioids is rare and respiratory depression is only a concern when the patient is first introduced to the opioid. This problem is quickly overcome as the body becomes used to the presence of the opioid. Tolerance to the pain-reducing effects of the medication can also occur. Careful assessments should be made to avoid underdosing, which can cause pain to become out of control and unmanageable.

Tolerance and pseudo tolerance

Tolerance is the adaptation of the body to continued exposure to a drug or chemical. The effects of the drug at the same level of exposure are minimized over time. Additional dosing is required to maintain the same outcomes.

Pseudotolerance is the misguided perception of the health care provider that a patient's need for increasing doses of a drug is due to the development of tolerance when in reality disease progression or other factors are responsible for the increase in dosing needs.

Addiction and pseudoaddiction

Addiction is a primary and constant, neuro-biologic disease with genetic, psychosocial and environment factors that create an obsessive and irrational need or preoccupation with a substance. Addictive behaviors include unrestricted, continued cravings, compulsive and persistent use of a drug despite harmful experiences and side effect.

Pseudoaddiction is an assumption that the patient is addicted to a substance when in actuality the patient is not experiencing relief from the medication. It is prolonged, unrelieved pain that may be the result of under-treatment. This situation may lead the patient to become more aggressive in seeking medicated relief, thus resulting in the inappropriate "drug seeker" label.

Physical dependence

Physical dependence is a state of bodily adaptation to the presence of a drug or other substance. This adaptation is manifested by a specific withdrawal syndrome that can be produced by abrupt cessation, rapid dose reduction, decreased blood level of the drug, and/or administration of an antagonist. The resulting symptoms are negative and can include increased heart rate and blood pressure, sweating, and tremors. Serious withdrawal consequences include confusion, seizures, and visual hallucinations. While the body has compensated for the presence of the substance, it may or may not be manifested in the patient's thinking and other psychosocial factors.

Outcome indicators for pain control in the palliative care setting

Effective pain control in the palliative care setting begins with the initial evaluation. The goal of palliative care is to bring any pain that is not well controlled within the patient's own comfort level within the first 48 hours. From this point, pain control should be maintained within these parameters with provisions for breakthrough pain episodes and changes in overall pain levels. Pain that is out of control should be managed by active intervention within a predetermined time limit. It is the mission of palliative care to improve the overall quality of the patient's life. In turn, no patient should face death or die in the presence of uncontrolled pain. Adverse effects should be anticipated and prevented whenever possible. When adverse effects occur, they should also be treated in the same timely manner.

Conscious sedation

Conscious sedation is identified as a minimally depressed state of awareness in which the patient maintains the ability to respond appropriately to verbal and physical stimulus and commands. Patients are also capable of maintaining their own airways, as well as continuing to protect themselves with reflexive responses. Conscious sedation is maintained with analgesics and sedatives in order perform various medical and surgical procedures. This procedure must be used with precaution in order to prevent loss of consciousness. In case of this type of emergency, health care personnel should have equipment on hand for airway management, resuscitation, and medications for sedation reversal, such as naloxone and benzodiazepines.

Patient Care: Symptom Management

Indications of swallowing disorder

Early warning signs may include changes in eating habits or attitudes. The patient may become impulsive in regard to eating, show inattention or signs of "playing" with their food during eating episodes, refuse to eat in the presence of others, or avoid certain previously enjoyed foods or liquids. Meal times and postures while eating may change. The patient may begin using large amounts of fluid to wash down solids, begin taking smaller bites or laboriously chewing them, and then take several swallows following each bite with frequent throat clearing. Otherwise unexplained weight loss may occur. If oral-pharyngeal dysfunction is present, the speech may become slurred and imprecise. The voice may sound "wet." Assessment may show a dry mouth with thick secretions coating the tongue and palate, and residual food may be present. Secretion drooling or leakage of liquids may also occur. More advanced signs include coughing and choking while attempting to eat, nasal regurgitation, and aspiration.

Interventions helpful for expressive aphasia

Expressive aphasia is also known as Broca aphasia. Patients with expressive aphasia are able to understand what is being said to them and they also know what they want to say, but they are unable or limited in their ability to speak. Provide an unhurried and attentive atmosphere when initiating communication with the expressive aphasic patient. Remove distractions and external stimulus as much as possible and speak in a normal tone using simple, direct phrasing to help avoid misunderstandings. A communication board is helpful to them and allows them to show their thoughts rather than speak them. Eye blinking responses to simple yes/no types of questions can be useful in locked-in conditions where the patient maintains comprehension but also has extremely limited neuromuscular function.

Dysphagia

Dysphagia is difficultly swallowing any substance. This difficulty also affects airway protection and patient safety. Food may become caught in the upper digestive tract or be diverted into the trachea causing aspiration, choking and possible asphyxiation. It can be both frightening and discouraging to the patient. Posture modifications such as tucking in the chin or tilting the head may help promote food movement along the upper digestive tract. Changes can also be made to the texture and consistency of the food. Artificial saliva can also help make swallowing easier. It is also possible to bypass the upper digestive tract and introduce nutrients as gastrostomy or jejunostomy tubal feedings for those patients who desire such intervention.

Myoclonus

Myoclonus presents as sudden, uncontrollable, nonrhythmic jerking of the extremities. This jerking can be induced by tapping on the affected muscle group. Early identification and rapid treatment are critical. Myoclonus can be exhausting for the palliative care patient and can progress to more severe neurological dysfunction, including seizures. Though the precise cause is unknown, myoclonus is often a result of opioids given in high doses, particularly in patients with renal failure. Other reported causes of myoclonus include brain surgery, intrathecal catheter placement, AIDS dementia, and hypoxia. Nocturnal myoclonus (nonrhythmic jerking of the extremities just prior to sleep) is common and often precedes opioid-induced myoclonus. Opioid rotation and use of adjuvants to reduce the amount of opioid needed are the primary treatments.

Status epilepticus

Status epilepticus is a seizure lasting longer than 5 minutes, or the state of repeated seizures without a subsequent return to consciousness, or return of normal brain function, between each separate episode. Status epilepticus is considered to be a neuro-oncological emergency. Treatment for status epilepticus focuses on maintaining a clear airway, protecting the patient from eminent harm, and administering medication in an attempt to resolve the episodes. Assess for adequate patient perfusion, give a glucose solution, evaluate the electrolytes, and administer IV benzodiazepines followed by IV phenytoin. Lorazepam is generally the first line of defense; however, if the seizure does not respond to treatment within the first 5 to 7 minutes, phenytoin or fosphenytoin should be added. In extreme cases, barbiturates, anesthesia, neuromuscular blocks, and propofol may be needed to control seizure activity.

Causes of seizures in palliative care patients

Careful assessment must be done in the presence of seizures; there are multiple causes that should be considered in the end-of-life patient. Assessment for these causes and new seizure activity should be included in all patients, whether actual seizures have been present to that point or not, in order to prevent them wherever possible. Seizures may be a preexisting disorder or new in onset. Primary or metastatic cancers to the brain are common causes. Medications, including phenothiazines, butyrophenones, tricyclic antidepressants, metabolites such as normeperidine, or the disruption of a drug the body has become physically dependent upon, such as benzodiazepines, preservatives, antioxidants, or other additives in the chemical formulas can also introduce new-onset seizures. Additional causes include HIV, infection, metabolic disorders, stroke, hemorrhage, and oxygen deprivation. Though less frequent, some rare paraneoplastic disorders may also be possible causes.

Treatment options for active seizures in terminally ill patients

The most common anticonvulsant medications used to treat seizures are diazepam, lorazepam, midazolam, phenytoin, and phenobarbital. If the possibility of seizures exists, the first line of defense is generally lorazepam as-needed. Lorazepam can be given intravenously or in a solution of intensol sublingually. The medication chosen may also depend on drug availability, practitioner knowledge and comfort base, and the delivery routes available with a given patient. When the oral route cannot be used, diazepam and phenobarbital can be given intramuscularly. Diazepam is also available as a rectal gel. Phenobarbital is available in a parenteral solution and for oral and rectal administration. Fosphenytoin is an option for subcutaneous delivery but has a greater cost. Intravenous phenytoin also carries serious complications, including edema, discoloration, and pain, referred to as the "purple glove syndrome."

Early signs of spinal cord compression

Back pain is the primary symptom of spinal cord compression. It generally presents as pain that increases when lying flat and improves when standing. The patient may also complain of bowel or bladder changes, leg weakness, or a "funny feeling" in the legs. These symptoms need to be recognized and treated immediately to prevent paralysis. Pain may be present long before any neurological dysfunction is detected. Patients presenting with localized back pain and a normal neurological examination may still be experiencing as much as 75% spinal cord compression. In a patient with cancer, back pain is presumed to be cord compression, until proven otherwise, and treated as a medical emergency. This may help to prevent permanent loss of function. The use of steroids, surgical decompression, or hormone and radiation therapy can decrease the pain and usually preserve function. Steroids alone may decrease pain and preserve function for those in the last stages of life that do not want any form of radiation therapy. Neurological function must be assessed before starting therapy in order to gauge responsiveness

Edema

Edema is a result of excess fluid gathering within the tissues (interstitially). Capillary filtration exceeds lymph drainage, creating a fluid imbalance. The resulting fluid retention causes swelling, decreased skin mobility, tightness, tingling, decreased strength, mobility, and discomfort ranging from aching to severe pain. Skin can change color or even burst from the pressure. Edema is generally assessed according to the pitting scale.
- 1+ edema means the fluid buildup is barely detectable.
- 2+ edema shows a slight indentation when pressed upon.
- 3+ edema shows a deep indentation for 5 to 30 seconds when pressure is applied.
- 4+ edema creates a depression that is 1½ to 2 times greater than normal.

Edema treatment generally has good results when addressed in a timely manner. Left untreated, edema can transition to lymphedema.

SVCS

Superior vena cava syndrome (SVCS) is the result of a partial occlusion of the superior vena cava, which results in decreased venous blood flow from the head and neck to the right atrium. The blockage may result from cancerous growths. This is considered an emergency condition marked by headache, facial edema, hoarseness, dyspnea, and swollen arms. In rapid onset, the loss of circulation can be life-threatening. The severity and timing of symptom onset can be gradual or acute. Patients may report subtle signs such as swelling in the morning hours or increasing discomfort with bending forward or stooping. The most common complaint is dyspnea. Other physical findings can include vein distention in the neck and chest, a ruddy complexion or cyanosis, tachypnea, stridor, orthopnea, hoarseness, nasal stuffiness, or periorbital and conjunctival edema. As symptoms progress, mental status changes will occur, progressing from a stupor, coma, and seizures until the time of death.

Pericardial effusion

Pericardial effusion is defined as an accumulation of fluid or tumor cells within the pericardial sac. Effusions will affect nearly 20% of patients with lung cancer during the advanced stages of the disease. It is also associated with breast cancer, leukemia, and lymphoma. This condition carries a poor prognosis for these patients. Pericardial effusion can be caused by cancerous cells, the treatments used for malignancies, as well as nonmalignant causes. Other identifying causes include pericarditis, congestive heart failure, uremia, myocardial infarction, autoimmune diseases, infections, hypothyroidism, and renal and hepatic failure. Clinical signs and symptoms are dependent on the amount of fluid, how quickly it accumulates, and the general health of the cardiac tissue. Dyspnea is the most common presenting symptom; the patient may be unable to speak more than one word with each breath. There are also complaints of chest heaviness, dry cough, and generalized weakness. Physically, tachycardia is present as the body tries to compensate for the reduced cardiac output.

Angiogenesis

Angiogenesis is the normal physiological process in which new blood vessels grow from preexisting vessels. This process is part of normal wound healing; however, is it is also a key component in creating tumors that mutate from a benign state to a malignant state. There are three main types of angiogenesis: sprouting, intussusceptive, and therapeutic. Sprouting angiogenesis sends proliferating endothelial cells out from the tumor, acting much like roots, trying to capture new areas for cell growth. Intussusceptive tumors are also identified as "splitting." The original capillary walls split into two, forming new, separate cells. Therapeutic angiogenesis represents the body's natural defenses in order to help combat disease or tissue repair. Tumors use angiogenesis in order to expand and spread the tumor in the process of metastasis. Angiogenesis research expects to identify ways to inhibit this process in the tumor cells.

Congestive heart failure

Congestive heart failure is the inability of the heart to function properly. It may affect the right ventricle, left ventricle, or both. Coronary artery disease is the most common cause. Symptoms can include weight gain, peripheral edema in the feet and ankles with possible pitting, nocturia, decreased urine output, shortness of breath including nocturnal dyspnea, wheezing, cough, distended neck veins, heart palpitations or irregular heartbeat, anxiety, restlessness, cyanosis or pallor, fatigue, weakness, and fainting. Auscultation may also reveal heart murmurs or extra heart sounds, crackles in the lungs or decreased breath sounds, and an enlarged liver. Occasionally, the disease process may be silent and only manifest during times of infection with high fever, anemia, arrhythmias, hyperthyroidism, and kidney disease.

Dyspnea

Pathophysiological mechanisms
The vascular bed begins to decrease from thromboemboli, tumor emboli, vascular obstruction, radiation, chemotherapy toxicity, or concomitant emphysema. As the vascular bed decreases, the physiological dead space causes increased ventilation demands. This results in hypoxemia and severe deconditioning with metabolic acidosis and alterations in carbon dioxide output (VCO_2) and arterial partial pressure of carbon dioxide (PCO_2). This also increases neural reflex activity, anxiety, and depression. Inspiratory muscle weakness from cachexia, electrolyte imbalances, neuromuscular abnormalities and steroid use, pleural or parenchymal disease, reduced chest wall compliance, and airway obstruction (such as asthma, tumor growth and COPD) can produce impaired mechanical responses and ventilatory pump impairment.

Symptom management
Dyspnea is the subjective sensation of breathlessness, or an inability to obtain the needed amount of air. It will occur in the majority of advanced cancer patients. Assessment for an underlying cause, if unknown, is appropriate and helps focus treatment. Dyspnea can be relieved by a high Fowler's position or leaning forward with the patient's arms supported on a table or other firm surface. Cool, moving air can be comforting and provide a peaceful, calming atmosphere. The patient may be prompted to perform previously learned relaxation techniques and pursed-lip breathing. Oxygen may be given, even in the nonhypoxemic patient, in an attempt to provide physical and

psychological comfort. However, oxygen treatment itself may be ineffective. Opioids, tranquilizers, and anxiolytics may also be administered as needed.

<u>Risk factors in the elderly palliative care patient</u>
Risk factors for dyspnea can include structural deviations such as a decrease in skeletal muscle, barrel chest, increased anteroposterior chest wall diameter with decreased chest wall elasticity, and decreased in alveoli elasticity. These factors increase the work of breathing while decreasing the maximum volume expiration and vital capacity. Other factors that can contribute to dyspnea include anemia, cachexia, dehydration, dry mucous membranes, thick secretions causing mucus plugs, ascites, fever with a reduced immune and febrile response, and decreased white blood cell count. Patients with heart failure, immobility, obesity, recent stomach, pelvic, or chest surgery, and lung diseases are at increased risk. There is also an increased risk for aspiration, deep vein thrombosis, and pulmonary embolism.

<u>BREATHES Program</u>
The BREATHES Program for management of dyspnea in the elderly palliative care patient is described below:
- B- Bronchospasm: Consider the use of albuterol nebulizers and/or steroids.
- R- Rales/crackles: If rales or crackles are present, fluid intake should be reduced by fluid restriction and discontinuation of IV therapy. Consider using diuretics at a dosage of 20 to 40 mg/day for furosemide or 100 mg daily of spironolactone.
- E- Effusion: Determine the presence of a pleural effusion by physical examination and chest x-ray. Treatments options such as thoracentesis or chest tube should be considered.
- Airway obstruction: Assess for aspiration risk and provide preventative measures, such as pureed meals, thickened liquids, and keeping the patient upright during and after meals.
- T- Tachypnea and breathlessness: Opioid use may reduce the respiratory rate and create feelings of breathlessness and anxiety. Frequent medication assessment is advised, including treatments for anxiety as needed. Providing cool, moving air may also help reduce feelings of breathlessness.
- H- Hemoglobin: If the hemoglobin is low, consider a blood transfusion.
- E- Education: Educate and support the patient and family.
- S- Secretions: If secretions are copious, provide pharmacological treatment.

Pleural effusion

A pleural effusion occurs when there is a discrepancy between the secretion and absorption of fluid in the pleural space. Secretion rates are increased and/or fluid absorption becomes restricted, causing excessive fluid to collect. The onset of a pleural effusion can be slow or rapid. The patient will most often present with dyspnea. Dyspnea generally results from the collapse of the lung due to the increased pleural fluid pressure. The inability to expand the lung leads to the complaints of dyspnea. As the affected area increases, dyspnea distress also increases, along with orthopnea and tachypnea, anorexia, malaise, and fatigue. The patient may also complain of a dry, nonproductive cough and an aching, heaviness, or dull pain in the chest. Treatment of a pleural effusion is palliative and symptomatic in nature, and is dependent on the surrounding circumstances, the overall patient condition, and proximity to death.

Hemoptysis

Hemoptysis is the expectoration of blood from the lower respiratory tract. It occurs frequently in patients with advanced cancer because of metastasis or infection. An additional common cause in the United States is bronchitis. Initial assessment needs to distinguish from gastrointestinal and nasopharyngeal bleeding. Patient complaints include cough, dyspnea, wheezing, chest pain, fever, night sweats, and weight loss. The severity of hemoptysis is determined by the amount of blood produced within a 24-hour period. Mild hemoptysis is the production of less than 15 to 20 mL of blood within that time period. Moderate hemoptysis requires expectoration of greater than 20 mL but less than 200 mL. Massive hemoptysis is 200 to 600 mL of blood expectorated within a 24-hour period. Massive hemoptysis occurs in fewer than 5% of cases but it is life-threatening and associated with an 85% mortality rate. The primary risk is asphyxiation from blood clots in the airway.

Therapy for PCP

Pneumocystis carinii pneumonia (PCP) is one of the most opportunistic infections and a common cause of pulmonary disease in individuals with HIV infection. The following are recommended treatments:

- Trimethoprim-sulfamethoxazole (TMP-SMX) is the recommended initial therapy for *Pneumocystis carinii* pneumonia treatment. Used in combination with corticosteroids, survival rates and treatment outcomes are greatly improved. It can also be used for prophylaxis treatment in adults experiencing immunosuppressive disease states, such as AIDS; this has had very positive results. Treatment can begin in the presence of a CD4+ count of less than 200 or oropharyngeal candidiasis.
- Dapsone is another choice for alternative therapy but it is uncommon and generally not preferred.
- Pentamidine or clindamycin are second-line therapy if the first-line therapy failed.

CF

Cystic fibrosis is a genetic disease that is eventually fatal. Care during the lifetime of the child with CF is focused on preventative measures to avoid disease complications. Therapeutic care for lung disease progression and palliative care for symptom management are also provided. Symptoms can present in the lungs, pancreas, urogenital system, skeleton, and skin. COPD and lung infections, deficient pancreatic enzymes, osteoporosis, and sweat that shows a high electrolyte concentration are signature complications. Symptoms and complications can include nasal polyposis, bronchiectasis, bronchitis, pneumonia, respiratory failure, gallbladder disease, intussusception, meconium ileus, salt depletion, nutritional malabsorption, pancreatitis, peptic ulcer, rectal prolapse, diabetes, arthritis, failure to thrive, and delayed puberty. Medical research continues to make progress that is extending the life of children with CF into their 20s, 30s, and occasionally into the 40s. Treatment includes control and prevention of infection. Treatment for excessive secretions and pulmonary complications is provided, as well as careful dietary monitoring.

Tuberculosis

Tuberculosis is common among immunosuppressed patients. Physical symptoms include night sweats, unexplained weight loss, and fatigue. Pulmonary tuberculosis also shows a chronic cough with active sputum production. If left untreated, tuberculosis may also spread to other organs and cause neurological diseases such as meningitis, bone infections, and urinary bleeding. A positive tuberculin skin test signifies a previous exposure to tuberculin organisms. However, it cannot pinpoint a recent change from a negative status unless the positive test is a follow-up to previous negative test results. The skin test alone cannot accurately pinpoint the time of exposure. An initial tuberculosis diagnosis for the presence of an active disease state can be obtained by finding acid-fast bacilli in stained smear samples from sputum or other body fluids. The initial diagnosis is confirmed by isolating *Mycobacterium tuberculosis* on culture or rapid nucleic acid test probes.

End stage respiratory disease

Regardless of the original underlying diagnosis, signs and symptoms, as well as their treatment, will be the same by the end stages. Profound dyspnea severely impacts the activities of daily living with frequent exacerbations and increasing use of emergency treatments. There is an increased respiratory infection and failure rate as the disease progresses. Respiratory failure results from a decreased PO_2 and increased PCO_2, which creates a carbon dioxide narcotic-like effect that suppresses the respiratory drive and causes a slow loss of consciousness until there is a complete stop of respirations. Increased stress in the lungs creates increased stress on the heart and may lead to lower peripheral edema, pulmonary hypertension, and right-sided heart failure. Fatigue and limited tolerance for activity, poor quality of life, weight loss, tachycardia, tachypnea, pneumonia, pneumothorax, and polycythemia are all common complications as well. Patients with a FEV_1 (forced expiratory volume at 1 second) of less than 0.75 L have a 30% chance of dying within 1 year

Constipation in palliative care patients

Primary or metastasized cancers directly affecting the bowel or pelvic area can cause intestinal obstruction or adhesions. Disease processes such as diabetes, hypothyroidism, hypokalemia, diverticular disease, hemorrhoids, colitis, and chronic neurological diseases can cause constipation. Hypercalcemia with related nutrition and appetite changes, decreased fluid intake, weakness, inactivity, confusion, depression, and changes in toileting habit can all slow motility. Medications such as opioids suppress motility and increase sphincter tone, as well as increase electrolyte and water absorption. Other medications that can cause constipation include anticholinergics, tricyclic antidepressants, antiparkinsonian drugs, iron, antihypertensives, antihistamines, antacids, and diuretics. Vinca alkaloid chemotherapy also causes constipation by damaging the myenteric plexus of the colon, causing increased contractions without increased movement.

Foods and medications to avoid to treat cancer-related diarrhea

Diarrhea-causing foods include high-fiber or gas-causing products such as legumes, raw vegetables, whole-grains, and popcorn. High-fat or heavily spiced foods may also cause difficulties. Milk and dairy products can be main offenders as well as caffeine or carbonated and high sugar or sorbitol drinks such as coffee, colas, prune, pear, cherry, peach, apple, and orange juices. High-risk foods, such as sushi, and food from street vendors, and buffets should be avoided.
Side effects from medications can also cause diarrhea. Standard culprits include antibiotics, laxatives, and medications containing magnesium or motility agents and stool softeners. Herbal supplements should not be overlooked. Milk thistle, aloe, cayenne, saw palmetto, and Siberian ginseng are often intestinal stimulants as well.

Nursing interventions to manage diarrhea

Assess the patient's environment for ease of care during the episode of diarrhea. Assess patient history for the duration and frequency of episodes, fluid and fiber intake, appetite, presence of nausea or vomiting, surgical and radiation therapy, presence of bacterial, protozoan, or viral diseases associated with diarrhea, as well as disease states associated with diarrhea to determine the most appropriate treatment methods. Physically assess the perineum or ostomy site for skin breakdown, fissures or hemorrhoids, and for impaction. The abdomen should be assessed for distention or the presence of palpable stool within the bowel. Evaluate the stool for signs of bleeding and for dehydration. Ensure that the perineum or stoma area is cleaned gently and thoroughly after each movement. Offer sitz baths as appropriate. Encourage small, frequent, bland meals with increased fluid intake. A low-residue diet with potassium-rich foods and homeopathic methods such as ginger tea, glutamine, and peeled apples may also be helpful.

Malignancy related types of ascites

Central ascites results from compression of the portal venous or lymphatic system compression from tumor invasion. With this process, there is a decrease in pressure as a result of limited protein intake and the catabolic state associated with cancer. Peripheral ascites results from deposits of tumor cells on the parietal or visceral peritoneum; the blockage occurs at this level rather than in the liver parenchyma. The presence of macrophages increases capillary permeability and contributes to increasing fluid retention. Mixed-type ascites is a combination of both peripheral and central ascites. Chylous malignant ascites occurs when cancer cells invade the retroperitoneal space, causing lymph flow obstruction for the lymph nodes or pancreas. Malignant ascites generally has a poor prognosis. Tumor cells make it difficult to reduce fluid accumulation. Cancers most often associated with ascites include ovarian, endometrial, breast, colon, gastric, and pancreatic cancer. Less common sources include mesothelioma, non-Hodgkin lymphoma, and prostate cancer.

Medical treatments of ascites

Central ascites and mixed-type ascites are associated with renal sodium and water retention, which indicates a treatment including restricted sodium and fluid intake may be beneficial in reducing the amount of fluid retention. Spironolactone is the preferred medication with a dosage of 100 to 400 mg/day. Furosemide 40 to 80 mg/day may also be helpful in initiating diuresis; be careful not to remove more fluid than is beneficial. Dehydration from overuse of furosemide can lead to electrolyte imbalances, hepatic encephalopathy, and prerenal failure. With mixed-type ascites, other dietary changes may also be needed. These can include a decreased fat intake and increased medium-chain triglycerides; shorter fatty acid chains may be easier to digest. Those with refractory ascites and a shortened life expectancy can benefit from the use of paracentesis. This treatment may also be helpful for tense ascites associated with cirrhosis or nonmalignant ascites. The removal of 4 to 6 liters per day has been deemed safe and effective with albumin infusion to prevent hypovolemia and renal impairment. Peritoneovenous shunts such as Denver or LeVeen are helpful for 75% to 85% of patients with nonmalignant ascites.

Nursing interventions for patients with ascites

Management of ascites involves understanding the underlying cause and focusing treatment to those specific needs. Fluid and sodium restrictions may help reduce the severity of ascites. This requires education for the patient and caregivers on the diet parameters and the expected outcomes for improved quality of life. The patient who faces the difficult cycle of thirst, hydration, and increased discomfort has a better chance of compliance with education and understanding of the mechanism of ascites. Supportive care such as comfort interventions, pillow supports, and loose clothing can be helpful. Good assessment skills and skin care to monitor and prevent skin breakdown are also essential. Recurring ascites may require repeated paracentesis. Helping the patient recognize the risk and benefit ratio of repeated paracentesis may become necessary.

Intractable hiccups

Intractable hiccups can occur from phrenic nerve or diaphragmatic irritation, distention of the stomach, chest or abdominal surgery, or metabolic disorders such as hyponatremia and intracerebral lesions. These conditions cause a spasmodic closure of the glottis at varying intervals. This closure results in the intermittent lowering of the diaphragm, which causes sharp inspiration and a corresponding sound generally known as a hiccup. Chlorpromazine in a dose of 25 mg by mouth or rectum three times a day is recommended for treatment of intractable hiccups caused by stress to the diaphragm from chemical, mechanical, or neurological irritation. In extreme cases, anesthetization of the phrenic nerve may be needed.

Nonpharmacological interventions for hiccups

Multiple treatments for hiccups exist based on the physiological needs of the patient. Respiratory intervention include the classic method of breath holding as well as rebreathing into a paper bag, providing diaphragm compression, or stimulating the sneeze or cough reflex with spices or inhalants. Ice may also be placed in the mouth. Nasal and pharyngeal stimulation also includes a few well know "cures" such as drinking from the far side of a glass, eating a spoonful of sugar, or holding the nose and applying pressure. Stimulant inhalation may prove effective, as well as tongue traction, eating soft bread, drinking peppermint water to soothe the esophagus, or stimulating the palate with bitters such as cotton-tipped applicators soaked in lemon. Stimulation of the vagal nerve may be achieved through ocular compression, digital rectal massage, or careful carotid massage. Gastric distention relief can be achieved through fasting, the placement of a nasogastric tube to relieve abdominal distention, lavage, or vomiting. Psychiatric treatments include distraction and behavior modification techniques. Other miscellaneous methods include bilateral radial artery compression and acupuncture.

Pharmacological agents to treat hiccups

The following are pharmacological agents that may be used to treat hiccups:
- Simethicone 15 to 30 mL and metoclopramide 10 to 20 mg to reduce gastric distention.
- Baclofen 5 to 10 mg and midazolam 5 to 10 mg are effective muscle relaxants.
- Gabapentin 300 to 600 mg, carbamazepine 200 mg, and valproic acid 5 to 15 mg may be used as anticonvulsive agents.
- Dopamine agonists include haloperidol 1 to 5 mg and chlorpromazine 5 to 50 mg.
- Calcium channel blockers including phenytoin 200 to 300 mg, nefopam 10 mg, lidocaine 2 mg/min, quinidine 200 mg, and nifedipine 10 to 80 mg may also be used.
- Other medication choices include dexamethasone 40 mg, mephenesin 1,000 mg, amitriptyline 25 to 90 mg, methylphenidate 5 to 20 mg, and sertraline 50 mg.

Effects of nausea and vomiting on quality of life

As with any illness, the presence of nausea and vomiting has a negative effect on all aspects of the patient's well-being. Nausea and vomiting cause nutritional loss resulting in fluid and electrolyte imbalance, fatigue, and reduced ability of patients to care for themselves. These conditions place increased stress upon the patient and can result in distress, anxiety, fear, or loss of happiness and enjoyment. Lives and relationships are interrupted with a decrease in affection or sexual function and an increased dependence on the caregiver. It also increases the burden and stress in the caregiver and patient relationship. This condition may also increase the patient's fears related to the illness and the suffering it causes, including the spiritual meaning of the illness as a punishment for past deeds.

Antiemetics

The following are the 10 classes of drugs currently used as antiemetics:
1. Butyrophenones (haloperidol, droperidol) are used for opioid, chemical, and mechanical induced nausea.
2. Prokinetic agents (metoclopramide, domperidone) are used for gastric stasis and ileus.
3. Cannabinoids (dronabinol) are second-defense antiemetics that are more effective in young adults.
4. Phenothiazines (prochlorperazine, thiethylperazine, trimethobenzamide) are generally used for nausea and vomiting.
5. Antihistamines (diphenhydramine, cyclizine) are for intestinal obstruction, peritoneal irritation, and increased intracranial pressure (ICP).
6. Anticholinergics (scopolamine) are for intestinal obstruction, peritoneal irritation, increased secretions, and increased ICP.
7. Steroids (dexamethasone) can be used alone or as an adjuvant therapy.
8. Benzodiazepines (lorazepam) are most effective for nausea and vomiting aggravated by anxiety.
9. 5-HT_3 receptor antagonists (ondansetron, granisetron) are effective for chemotherapy, radiation therapy, and postoperative nausea and vomiting.
10. The somatostatin analog octreotide acetate can help with nausea and vomiting with intestinal obstruction. The anticholinergic dimenhydrinate is used for nausea and vomiting associated with dizziness and motion sickness.

Nonpharmacological self-care activities to treat nausea and vomiting

Preventative measure can be taken to help avoid nausea and vomiting episodes. Provide fresh air with a fan or open window but limit sights, sounds, and noxious smells that may precipitate the individual's nausea and vomiting. Patients should avoid consuming sweet, salty, fatty, and spicy foods. Food should be bland and served at room temperature or cold. The patient should be instructed to wear loose-fitting clothes during meal times. Fluid consumption with meals should be restricted to just the amount needed to ease the passage of food. Instruct the patient to reduce the quantity of food consumed at one time by eating smaller, more frequent meals, and lying down for up to 2 hours after eating. Application of a cool, damp cloth to the forehead, neck, and wrists may also help fight nausea. If vomiting does occur, reinforce the need for oral care after each episode both for relief of unpleasant sensory side effects and for general oral health.

Nonpharmacological interventions to combat nausea and vomiting

Nonpharmacological interventions that may be used to help combat nausea and vomiting are discussed below:
- *Self-hypnosis:* Involves invoking an altered state of consciousness in anticipation of nausea and vomiting episodes to decrease frequency, severity, amount, and duration of uncomfortable episodes.

- *Relaxation:* Progressive relaxation of muscle groups often involving imagery, which may be helpful in conjunction with chemotherapy-induced nausea and vomiting.
- *Biofeedback:* Electromyographic or skin temperature controlled responses to changes within the body. It may be used with relaxation during chemotherapy.
- *Imagery:* Mentally removing the focus from unpleasant side effects and refocusing the mind on other images. It increases self-control while decreasing length and perceptions of nausea and vomiting episodes.
- *Distraction:* Diverting attention to other activities such as video games, puzzles, or humor.
- *Desensitization:* Involves relaxation and visualization to decrease perceptions of nausea and vomiting.
- *Acupressure:* A form of massage to increase energy flow and improve emotion.
- *Music therapy:* Often used with other therapies to influence physiological, psychological, and emotional states during and after nausea and vomiting episodes.

Stomatitis

Stomatitis is an inflammation of the oral cavity, including the lips, tongue, and mucous membranes. This inflammation may be associated with conditions such as viral infections, chemical irradiation, chemotherapy, radiation therapy, mouth breathing, medication side effects, paralysis of nerves supplying the oral cavity, or area irritation or trauma such as sun damage or irritation from foreign bodies. Nasal catheters used to provide oxygen and nutrition therapies and endobrachial tubes inserted for surgery increase the patient's vulnerability to stomatitis by irritation. Ill-fitting dental appliances can also cause irritation. Symptoms include patient complaints of oral pain with eating or drinking and difficulty swallowing. Physical manifestations include bad breath, oral lesions or ulcers, swollen cervical lymph nodes, possible fever, and mucous membranes that are easily damaged. Treatment depends on identifying and treating the underlying cause as well as comfort measures for symptomatic complaints. Mucous membranes need to be kept moist and clear from secretions. Careful oral care, including flossing and ongoing assessments for areas of damage, needs to be provided. Irritating items should be removed or carefully maintained. Systemic and topical analgesics can be used.

Ileus

An ileus is the cessation of peristalsis. The ileus itself is generally painless, but the loss of forward motion within the intestines can result in an intestinal obstruction, abdominal cramps, constipation, fecal vomiting, abdominal distention, and atrophy or collapse or surrounding intestines. Operative anesthesia and medications for pain control are common causes of an ileus. Postoperative ileus can be prevented by encouraging early ambulation and other activity. The use of nonopioids to control pain will prevent interference with bowel function. Oral intake should also be encouraged, even prior to the presence of bowel sounds. The ileus may resolve itself within 2 to 3 days with activity and oral intake. The patient should be monitored for fluid and electrolyte imbalances, blood pressure changes, and changes in abdominal girth. If the ileus is the result of another illness or treatment, care should focus on resolving this problem. Colonoscopy or a rectal tube may also aid in decompression.

Bowel strangulation, large bowel obstruction, and small bowel obstruction

The symptoms of bowel strangulation, large bowel obstruction, and small bowel obstruction are described below:

- *Bowel strangulation:* Severe, steady pain rather than cramping generally indicates that the blood supply has been completely cut off to an area of the intestines where there is an obstruction. This is considered a medical emergency.
- *Large bowel obstruction:* A large bowel obstruction usually causes cramping pains in the lower abdomen, below the level of the navel, that increase over time. There is a generalized feeling of bloating in the lower stomach and pelvic area. Either diarrhea or constipation may be present. Vomiting is not common.
- *Small bowel obstruction:* Symptoms of small bowel obstruction include cramping, colicky pains that come in waves in the middle to upper abdomen; these can generally be relieved with vomiting. Emesis is generally green in color. If left untreated, pain may become lessened over time as the bowel stops contracting. Constipation and an inability to pass gas are most common. Diarrhea and flatulence can occur with a partial obstruction. Patients will complain of feeling bloated. High-pitched stomach noises will decrease and stop as the bowl slows down.

Pureed, mechanically altered, and soft diet

Pureed, mechanically altered, and soft diet are defined below:

- Pureed: Foods are altered or processed in a blender to add liquid and change the consistency to smooth. A pureed diet is intended to reduce tongue function and the need for chewing. Pureed consistency foods include applesauce, yogurt, thin mashed potatoes, and puddings.
- Mechanically altered diet: Ground or finely chopped foods form small masses that require some, though minimal, chewing and tongue control. Possible foods include pasta, scrambled eggs, cottage cheese, and ground meats.
- Soft diet: Foods are not mechanically altered but chosen for their naturally soft qualities. These foods still require some chewing when presented in small pieces, but they also allow for reduced endurance and attention span. Foods include soft meats, canned fruits, and baked fish. Raw vegetables, bread, and tough meats should be avoided.

Potential complications of enteral support

Complications related to enteral nutritional support falls into four basic categories: aspiration, diarrhea, constipation, and dumping syndrome. Cases of aspiration may be caused by the use of a large-bore tube introducing formula too quickly or in too large of an amount. It is evidenced by fever and cough. Diarrhea or watery stools may result from the use of a hyperosmotic solution, an infusion rate that is too rapid, or lactose intolerance. Hard, infrequent stools result from inadequate supplemental fluid intake or inadequate fiber. Dumping syndrome can also result from the use of high-volume feeding boluses or hyperosmotic fluids, and can cause weakness, dizziness, nausea, palpitations, syncope, and diarrhea.

Agents used to decrease bladder contractility

Extended-release and transdermal agents include extended-release tolterodine 2 to 4 mg, trospium chloride 20 mg, extended-release oxybutynin 5 to 15 mg, and transdermal oxybutynin 3.9 mg.

Classic anticholinergics include propantheline 7.5 to 30 mg, immediate-release oxybutynin 7.5 to 15 mg, hyoscyamine (available as tablets or sublingual tablets) 0.125 to 0.375 mg, dicyclomine hydrochloride 10 to 20 mg, flavoxate 100 mg, and belladonna and opium suppositories. These medications work to decrease the frequency of urination urges and/or increase bladder capacity. Dry mouth, flushing, constipation, drowsiness, and blurred vision are common side effects for most of these medications. Pseudoephedrine and imipramine (tricyclic antidepressant) may also be useful for treating stress urinary incontinence.

DIAPERS mnemonic

The DIAPERS mnemonic describes the causes of acute urinary incontinence.
- D - Delirium: Acute delirium and the related confusion may cause urinary incontinence.
- I - Infection: A urinary tract infection can cause or worsen incontinence.
- A - Atrophic urethritis: Atrophic urethritis creates irritative voiding symptoms and stress incontinence.
- P - Pharmacy: Medications such as opioids, sedatives, antidepressants, antipsychotics, and antiparkinsonian drugs can reduce contractility and increase urinary retention, overflow, and stress incontinence.
- E - Excessive urine production: Chronic disease states such as diabetes mellitus cause polyuria and affect smooth muscle and nerve involvement.
- R - Restricted mobility: Immobility and restricted accesses to appropriate toileting facilities lead to urinary incontinence.
- S - Stool impaction: Stool impaction can result in urinary retention, urinary tract infection, and incontinence.

Medication options for hemorrhagic cystitis

The following are medication options for hemorrhagic cystitis:
- Aminocaproic acid with a loading dose of 5 g orally or parenterally followed by hourly doses of 1 to 1.25 g acts as a fibrinolysis inhibitor. It carries risks of clot retention and decreased blood pressure. This treatment may not be used in patients with upper urinary tract bleeding or vesicoureteral reflux. The time for treatment to take effect is 8 to 12 hours.
- Silver nitrate and alum (ammonium or potassium salt) in an irrigation solution, administered intermittently or continuously, causes chemical cauterization of the vessels. It may also cause functional obstruction or aluminum toxicity. Irrigation requires an average of 21 hours to complete the treatment process.
- Formalin (aqueous formaldehyde) acts to rapidly repair the bladder mucosa; however, this treatment is very painful and requires anesthesia. Formalin treatment may also cause fibrosis, papillary necrosis, fistula, or peritonitis.

Azotemia

Azotemia is a sign of renal failure. It represents abnormal levels of nitrogen-based compounds such as urea, and creatinine within the blood. This build-up is generally caused by insufficient filtering through the kidneys. Prerenal azotemia results from a lack of blood flow to the kidneys for filtering. Postrenal azotemia results from obstructed urinary flow. Other forms of azotemia may be caused by specific disease processes such as congestive heart failure, shock, severe burns, extensive vomiting and diarrhea, liver failure or trauma to the kidneys. Some antiviral medications can also cause azotemia. Signs and symptoms can include decreased urine output, fatigue, confusion or decreased awareness, pale skin, rapid pulse, dry mouth, complaints of thirst, edema and orthostatic blood pressure. Treatments for azotemia may be cause specific or include hemodialysis or peritoneal dialysis.

Asthenia

Asthenia is the medical term for a debilitating feeling of weakness without an actual loss of muscle strength. Weakness may be muscle-group specific or affect the entire body. Distinguishing between asthenia and actual muscle weakness can sometimes be difficult. Often, asthenia will progress to muscle weakness in the presence of chronic diseases. Asthenia is most commonly seen among patients suffering from chronic fatigue syndrome, sleep disorders, and chronic heart, lung, adrenal, and kidney diseases. It is also identified in conjunction with wasting diseases such as cancer and anemia. Common causes of asthenia in palliative care settings include Addison disease, anemia, anxiety, chemotherapy, chronic pain, dehydration and electrolyte imbalances, depression, diabetes, heart disease, infections, medications including narcotics, and paraneoplastic syndrome.

Xerostomia

Xerostomia is the sensation of a dry mouth. It can be experienced with or without decreased oral secretions. It may also be described as a burning or soreness of the oral tissues. Because of its common nature, it may be difficult to pinpoint an exact cause; it is often related to the interactions of multiple drugs, including antihistamines and anticholinergics. Other common causes include head and neck surgeries, chemotherapy and radiation, infection, inflammation, disease processes focused on the mouth and throat areas, immunocompromised conditions, dehydration, or various psychological factors, such as anxiety. Assessment and treatment are imperative to prevent further mouth and esophageal problems, such as dental caries, soft tissue irritations, lesions, and infections. Xerostomia can also cause bad breath, changes in taste, and swallowing and speech difficulties that can be frustrating and further complicating for the patient.

Alginate, enzymatic, semi-permeable film and hydrocolloid dressings

Alginate, enzymatic, semi-permeable film and hydrocolloid dressings are compared below:
- Alginate: An alginate dressing is best for wounds with heavy drainage. It controls secretions and reduces bacterial contamination. Pain is reduced by softening the surrounding tissues and reducing the pressure caused by excessive exudates. Alginate dressings are nonadherent and easily removed.
- Enzymatic dressings: An enzymatic dressing aids in loosening necrotic tissue. This treatment is appropriate for patients in long-term care or unable to sustain surgical/sharp debridement. Dressing changes do not tend to cause additional discomfort.
- Semipermeable film: Not absorbent and cannot be used when there is drainage present. It can help protect against early damage and assist with healing. The film minimizes pain by covering exposed nerve endings. However, because they adhere to the skin and wound bed, removal can be painful.
- Hydrocolloid dressings: Can only absorb small amounts of exudates. It is useful for mild debridement and keeps the wound bed moist to promote granulation. They can also assist with pain relief by minimizing exposure of the wound to air. Proper removal is required to decrease pain. Some are specifically designed for better attachment in the difficult sacral area.

Necessary assessment information in the presence of cutaneous malignancy

Does the location of the wound impair mobility or areas that are difficult to dress? Define the wound appearance in terms of size, color, tunneling, percentage of viable and necrotic tissues, bleeding and exudates, odor, and presence of infection. These affect the type of treatment and bandage types that may be needed. Assess the surrounding skin for redness, fragility, nodular, macerated, or radiation-related damage to determine the extent of tissue damage or metastasis. Is there itching or deep or superficial pain, including aching, stabbing, burning, or stinging, present? When is it most noticeable? Assess for potential complications from nearby major blood vessels, organs, or airway, creating the potential for hemorrhage, vessel obstruction, or a compromised airway.

Stages of pressure ulcers

The National Pressure Ulcer Advisory Panel developed a staging system to ensure that definitions for pressure ulcers were standardized.
- Stage I: Nonblanchable erythema Intact, reddened area that does not blanch. (Difficult to assess in darker skin). Area remains intact but the physical appearance is altered.
- Stage II: Partial thickness Destruction of the epidermis and/or dermis. This type of injury may be an intact blister, ruptured blister, or an open ulcer if it has a pinkish or a reddish wound bed.
- Stage III: Full thickness skin loss Epidermis and dermis have experienced loss and the injury now extends through to the subcutaneous fat tissue. Tunneling could be present. Muscle, tendons, and bones have not been injured.
- Stage IV: Full thickness tissue loss Damage has progressed to bone, muscle, or tendons. There is often tunneling present, osteomyelitis is common, and the depth of the ulcer will vary by location.
- Unstageable/Unclassified Injury is present and involves full thickness, but can not be staged until slough is removed.
- Suspected Deep Tissue Injury Discolored skin that is still intact but has been damaged. Suspect it is deeper than stage I, but the epidermis is still intact

Common locations of pressure ulcers

Pressure ulcers result from tissue compression and restricted blood flow to the affected area. Combined with moisture, shearing forces and friction result in tissue breakdown and necrosis. The most common sites for pressure ulcer occurrence are over areas with boney prominences or first points of contact when pressure is applied to a certain body area. Of these areas, the sacrum, greater trochanters or upper end of the femur, heels or calcaneus, and lateral and medial malleolus (protrusions around the ankle bone) are the most frequently affected. Other areas include the back of the head, scapula area, ischial tuberosities and hip, ribs and vertebrae, and the coccyx.

Bates-Jensen wound assessment tool

The Bates-Jensen wound tool rates various aspects of the wound on a scale. The higher the total score, the more severe the nature of the wound. Size is measured in centimeters, multiplying the length by the width. Depth is rated from 1 (noting tissue damage with intact skin covering) to 5 (involving supporting structures such as tendon and joint capsule). Edges are defined as indistinct, attached, not attached, rolled under, hyperkeratosis (callous-like), and fibrotic or scarred.

Undermining is assessed by using the tip of a cotton applicator around the edges of the wound to identify how far the wound extends under the visible edges. Necrotic tissue is labeled as white/gray nonviable, nonadherent yellow slough, loosely adherent yellow slough, adherent soft black eschar, or firmly adherent hard/black eschar. An amount of necrotic tissue is also noted. Exudate type (bloody, serosanguineous, serous, purulent, foul purulent) and amount (none, scant, small, moderate, large) are noted. The color of the surrounding tissue is assessed, as well as the presence of edema and pitting. Epithelialization and granulation are also noted.

Anxiety

Signs and symptoms
Anxiety is marked by feelings of excessive worry, irritability, restlessness, intense feelings of danger, and agitation. The source of the disquiet is unknown or very vague. Patients may have trouble falling or staying asleep and experience interference with other normal activities in their daily lives. Physically, the patient may be identified as having frequent crying spells, headaches, muscle tension, stomach and intestinal distress, palpitations, shortness of breath, or anorexia or overeating. Psychologically, the patient is vulnerable to unrealistic fears and obsessions with harmful ideas and compulsions. Patients may also try to self-medicate with multiple chemicals or substances in an attempt to alleviate these symptoms. An anxiety disorder is identified by the persistence of these symptoms over a period of 6 months or more.

Associated medical conditions
The physical root causes for anxiety can come from different sources.
- Cardiovascular: Hypovolemia, myocardial infarction (MI), paroxysmal atrial tachycardia (PAT), angina, congestive heart failure, and mitral valve prolapse.
- Endocrine disorders: Thyroid dysfunction, low or high blood sugar, Cushing disease, and carcinoid syndrome (excess secretion of serotonin, bradykinin, and other vasoactive chemicals).
- Metabolic: High potassium, high or low sodium levels, hyperthermia, anemia, and low blood sugar (hypoglycemia).
- Neoplasms: Islet cell adenomas, pheochromocytoma, a neural crest cell carcinoma.
- Neurological: Seizure disorders, vertigo, massive lesions, postconcussion syndrome, encephalopathy or generalized brain dysfunction, and general restlessness.
- Respiratory: Hypoxia, asthma, chronic obstructive pulmonary disease (COPD), pneumonia, pulmonary edema or embolus, respiratory distress.

Associated medications and other substances
Chemically induced anxiety can result from either the introduction of the substance or withdrawal from a substance that the body has become accustomed to. Everyday substances such as caffeine, decongestants, and antihistamines are known to increase anxiety. Alcohol and nicotine cause physical addictions. Their withdrawal is also associated with vague feelings of unease, discomfort, or dread associated with anxiety. Withdrawal from hypnotics causes anxiety. Benzodiazepines and their subsequent withdrawal can also cause anxiety. Other common medications include thyroid replacement formulas, neuroleptics, corticosteroids, bronchodilators, epinephrine, antihypertensives, antiparkinsonian medications, oral contraceptives, anticholinergics, anesthetics, and analgesics. Toxins and digitalis toxicity can cause anxiety. The street drugs marijuana and cocaine are also common causes.

Depression

Signs and symptoms
The depressed patient may present with any number of the following: depressed mood, insomnia or hypersomnia, an absence of pleasure in previously enjoyed activities, psychomotor retardation, fatigue, feelings of worthlessness and guilt, or an inability to concentrate, make decisions, or remember important information. The patient may experience significant and unexplained weight loss or weight gain. In severe cases, he or she may also disclose recurrent thoughts of death or suicide. Severity is assigned by the presence of an expressed intent with a plan and means to carry out a suicide attempt, as well as previous attempts. The hallmark symptoms of depression are appetite and sleep changes and decreased energy and concentration. However, in the presence of physical illness, these symptoms can be masked or created by the disease process or its treatments. With preexisting illness, symptoms such as fearfulness, depressed or changed appearance, social withdrawal, brooding, self-pity and pessimism, and a depressed mood or affect that cannot be changed or lifted may be more reliable indicators of depression.

Associated medical conditions
Patients experiencing depression have a greater tendency toward medical illnesses and vice versa. Underlying causes and links may be found in multiple areas of the assessment. Depression may be a risk factor for cardiovascular disease, congestive heart failure, arrhythmias, and heart attacks. Within the central nervous system, cerebral anoxia, cerebrovascular accident, Huntington disease, subdural hematoma, Alzheimer disease and dementia, HIV infection, carotid stenosis, temporal lobe epilepsy, multiple sclerosis, postconcussion syndrome, myasthenia gravis, narcolepsy, and subarachnoid hemorrhage patients are at increased risk. Other causes can include rheumatoid arthritis, thyroid disease, diabetes, Cushing disease, Addison disease, anemia, lupus, liver disease, syphilis, encephalitis, alcoholism, and general malnutrition.

Associated medications and substances
Chemically induced depression can result from either the introduction of the substance or withdrawal from a substance. Preexisting depression can be worsened in the presence of these substances. Everyday substances such as alcohol and analgesics are known to increase depression. Withdrawal from alcohol is also associated with vague feelings of unease, discomfort, or dread associated with depression and anxiety. Other common medications include hypoglycemic agents, steroids, chemotherapy, antimicrobials, L-dopa, antihypertensives, antiparkinsonian medications, oral contraceptives or other forms of estrogen and progesterone therapy, benzodiazepines, phenothiazines, amphetamines, lithium carbonate, heavy metals, and cimetidine.

Palliative nutrition

The patient receiving palliative care should be permitted to eat whatever he or she desires. Palliative nutrition should not focus on calories or content. The focus should be on the patient's desires and preferences. However, fatigue is a major concern for the palliative patient. Education should be provided about the importance of proper nutrition and adequate energy-providing foods. It may be helpful to recommend nutritious, high-protein, nutrient-dense foods as snacks. Small, frequent meals may also be preferable to large meals. Encourage adequate fluid intake as appropriate and frequent oral hygiene. As needed, the use of protein supplements may also be suggested.

Anorexia

Anorexia is defined as a lack or loss of appetite, or an inability to eat, with resulting weight loss. In the early stages, anorexia can usually be resolved, and any weight loss can be replaced, with increased intake. Unchecked, anorexia leads to protein-calorie malnutrition (PCM) and loss of fat tissue and lean muscle mass. These conditions are common in patients with advanced cancer, especially those directly related to the digestive system, and AIDS. Any number of things may contribute to or cause anorexia, including pain, loss of or change in taste, changed sensitivity to odors, loss of sense of smell, changes in sight, gastric dysfunction or malabsorption, nausea, vomiting, diarrhea, constipation or obstruction, infection, fever, change in metabolic rate, difficulty or loss of swallowing function, breathing restrictions, alcoholism, or chemical dependency.

Megestrol acetate

Megestrol acetate is a progestin and antineoplastic available as tablets or an oral suspension. It is used most often for breast and endometrial cancers, as well as an appetite stimulant. With breast cancer, a dosage of 40 mg four times a day is used. In endometrial cancer, this amount can be increased up to a total of 320 mg per day in evenly divided doses. For significant weight loss, megestrol acetate is normally given in doses of 400 mg twice daily. It can only be given to a level of 800 mg/day. The most common side effects of megestrol are increased appetite, fluid retention, and occasionally nausea. Often, any nausea will resolve itself within the first few weeks of taking the medication. Very rare allergic reactions may manifest, as well as jaundice or elevated blood pressure.

Cachexia

Cachexia is distinctly different from anorexia. The term cachexia is Greek in origin meaning "bad condition." It is defined as a state of general ill health and malnutrition, producing marked weakness and emaciation. It will occur in most patients with cancer and is the main cause of death in more than 20% of these patients. It is also common with AIDS, congestive heart failure, severe sepsis, tuberculosis, and other debilitating chronic illnesses. Anorexia can contribute to the development of cachexia; however, unlike anorexia, there is an equal loss of fat and muscle as well as a marked loss of bone mineral content in cachexia. It does not respond to nutritional supplements or increased intake. Cachexia develops from a systemic inflammatory response and metabolic imbalance in the presence of proinflammatory cytokines. The resulting catabolic state becomes self-reinforcing and continues to degrade the patient's quality of life.

Associated metabolic abnormalities

Metabolic changes, in response to inflammation and cytokine production, are common in cancer and AIDS patients. It appears that these changes represent the initiating event for cachexia. Major metabolic changes include decreased glucose tolerance, insulin resistance, decreased lipoprotein lipase activity, and negative nitrogen balance, decreased skeletal and lean muscle mass in the presence of increased energy expenditures. Other metabolic changes include increased glucose production and turnover, protein synthesis, fatty acid oxidation, serum lipid, and triglyceride levels. These are accompanied by decreased body glycogen mass, body lipid mass, and fat synthesis. Voluntary motor activity and energy stores and balance are quickly depleted during this wasting process. Serum glucose and insulin levels and nitrogen excretion remain unchanged.

Effects of dehydration on terminal patients

Dehydration is considered a natural part of the dying process; it is a loss of normal body water. Common causes include vomiting, diarrhea, decreased food and fluid intake, loss of thirst sensation, fever or increased metabolic needs, medications use such as diuretics that promote fluid loss, or renal complications that do not allow for proper clearance of excess liquid and electrolytes. Not treating dehydration can decrease cough and congestion, edema and ascites, and nausea and vomiting. The decrease in the frequency of urination that results from dehydration can actually improve the quality of life by reducing irritation and infection related to elimination treatments. However, dehydration can also aggravate confusion and restlessness. Patients at the end of life do not commonly experience thirst due to dehydration, and treatment can actually increase discomfort. Dry mouth is a common symptom of dehydration at the end of life and should be managed with comfort measures.

Complications from artificial hydration

The following are potential complications from various routes of artificial hydration:
- IV peripheral: The peripheral IV site should be monitored every few hours for the presence of pain, infiltration, infection, and phlebitis. Its usefulness is limited to a short duration.
- IV central: Though treatment duration is longer, the central IV carries increased risks for sepsis, hemothorax, pneumothorax, thrombosis from the central vein, catheter vein or catheter fragment, air embolus, brachial plexus injury, and arterial laceration.
- Hypodermoclysis: Injecting fluid into the subcutaneous space is a short-term option useful in the palliative care situation where oral or IV hydration cannot be achieved. It carries risks of pain, infection, volume overload and third spacing, tissue sloughing, localized bleeding, and electrolyte disturbances.

Initiating or continuing artificial fluids and hydration

The decision to begin artificial hydration is an easier task to follow through with than the decision to stop artificial fluids. Termination is a much more problematic and emotional decision. The decision to initiate artificial fluids is often made ahead of the perceived crisis, whereas the termination of hydration must be reached without the patient's direct input in most cases. Additionally, the psychological weight of death is not as pronounced when declining to initiate hydration efforts. Ethical, moral, and most religious viewpoints generally hold that there is no difference between withholding and withdrawal of hydration measures as it affects the individual's life and impending death. Consider the following criteria in determining hydration efforts:
- The overall effect on the quality of life.
- The patients' wishes and goals for the end of life.
- Discomforting symptoms that may be aggravated by hydration.
- The effects of hydration on the patient's level of consciousness.

Hydration limitations on the patient's well-being, mobility, interactions, stress levels, and finances must be considered.

Hyponatremic, hypernatremic, and isotonic dehydration

The symptoms of hyponatremic, hypernatremic, and isotonic dehydration are as follows:
- Hyponatremic dehydration: Hyponatremic dehydration is identified by volume depletion, anorexia, weight loss, nausea, and vomiting with taste alteration. Skin turgor is decreased, and mucus membranes are dry. Sweating is reduced. Orthostatic hypotension, lethargy, restlessness, delirium, seizures, confusion, stupor, and coma may result. Laboratory results include azotemia, disproportionate blood urea nitrogen as compared with creatinine, hyponatremia, hemoconcentration, urine osmolarity, and high sodium concentration.
- Hypernatremic dehydration: Symptoms include thirst, fever, fatigue and muscle weakness, and mental status changes. Serum sodium levels are increased.
- Isotonic dehydration: Isotonic dehydration is distinctly different. It produces psychological effects of morose, aggression, apathy, and demoralization, as well as a general lack of coordination. There are few or no laboratory abnormalities.

Hypercalcemia

Hypercalcemia is identified as the overabundance of ionized calcium in the blood. Hypercalcemia occurs in up to 10% of cancer patients. Individuals with breast cancer and multiple myeloma have the highest rates of occurrence. Additional causes include hyperparathyroidism, lithium therapy, vitamin D, vitamin A, or aluminum intoxication, hyperthyroidism, and milk-alkali syndrome. If left untreated, hypercalcemia can cause irreversible renal damage, coma, or death. Untreated hypercalcemia has a 50% mortality rate. Symptoms may vary depending on the amount of excess calcium. Presenting complaints are generally fatigue, lethargy, nausea, polyuria, and confusion. If left unchecked, the combination of nausea and polyuria can again increase the concentrations of calcium in the blood through dehydration. Additional symptoms include vomiting, anorexia, and constipation. An electrocardiogram will show evidence of a shortened QT interval and possible arrhythmias. Careful assessment should be made to avoid attaching symptoms to other disease processes in the already ill patient. Treatment may include hydration with saline, bisphosphonate, diuretics, and glucocorticoids in order to lower serum calcium levels.

Cancer-related fatigue

Causes for cancer-related fatigue may be physiologic or psychological in nature. Fatigue may be related to depression, pain, anemia related to iron deficiencies, bleeding, hemolysis, or a nutritional deficiency, sleeping disorders, fluid and electrolyte imbalances, hypocalcemia, hypothyroidism, hypoxia, infection, or overmedicating. Other metabolic disorder as well as neurological disorders may also contribute to the fatigue evidenced in cancer patients. Mood disorders may also include unresolved anxiety or fears concerning the disease process or treatments. An overall change and increase in the amount of stress experienced can lead to fatigue. Impaired thinking, including dementia, can cause confusion around timing of the day and the need for active rest. Treatment strategies focus on finding and resolving the underlying cause for fatigue whenever possible.

Consideration during fatigue assessment

Where in the body is the fatigue experienced? Fatigue may be focused upon the extremities, mental faculties, or total body. What is its severity? Does fatigue interfere with the patient's daily activities? How long have the symptoms lasted? What factors seem to aggravate the symptoms of fatigue? What methods seem to help alleviate the fatigue? Are any of the patient's current medications a contributing factor? Does a physical exam and general appearance present evidence of medically based reasons for, or resulting harm related to, fatigue? What are the patient's muscle strength and nerve responses? Do the patient's vital signs include irregularities such as low blood pressure and pulse, irregular heart rate, or fever? Is the patient oxygenated and balanced within their hormone levels, fluid, and electrolytes? What is the patient's current mood and activity level? Are these changed from previous states?

Predisposing factors leading to fatigue

Factors related to fatigue can be placed in the following three main categories: personal, disease-related, or treatment-related.
- Personal factors encompass age, household and personal demands, hormonal changes outside of the disease process, fear, depression, anxiety, spirituality, conflicts, unmet goals, culture and ethnicity, income and its stability, the living environment, and the patient's relationships with his or her support system and caregivers. These all affect the individual's stamina and overall well-being.
- Fatigue may also be related to the disease or treatment processes. The overall disease state including the presence of metastases can produce fatigue and an overall change in the energy level. This can be coupled with anemia, uncontrolled pain, sleep changes and interruptions, changes in bowel and bladder habits, cachexia, and dyspnea, which all play major roles.
- In addition, treatment-related factors can be responsible for fatigue. These effects may result from radiation, chemotherapy, medication, or permanent physiologic consequences of the treatment methods.

Diseases with highest risk of fatigue related complications

Below are the disease processes with the highest risk of complications due to fatigue:
- Cancer: Patients most often report fatigue as the most distressing symptom they experience. This can also be a side effect of treatment depending on the type they are receiving and the cancer stage.
- Coronary artery disease (CAD): CAD affects nearly 13 million Americans and remains the leading cause of death. There is significant fatigue related to many of these cases.
- Chronic fatigue syndrome (CFS): CFS is most common among women.
- Chronic obstructive pulmonary disease (COPD): Fatigue is the second most prevalent symptom associated with COPD. The most prevalent is shortness of breath.
- End-stage renal disease (ESRD): For patients treated with hemodialysis, fatigue rates are nearly 100%; with peritoneal dialysis, the rate is approximately 80%.
- HIV/AIDS: Fatigue is often a presenting symptom before diagnosis.
- Multiple sclerosis (MS): Fatigue is the most common and disabling symptom that has no widely accepted pharmacological treatment for MS patients at this time.
- Parkinson disease (PD): Studies are lacking for exact information about rates; however, most agree that rates are extremely high.

Pharmacological interventions for fatigue

The following are pharmacological interventions that can be used to help treat fatigue:
- Methylprednisolone appears to increase patient activity.
- Methylphenidate improves pain relief and somnolence in cancer patients. It also appears to reduce fatigue and increase cognitive function when combined with daily exercise.

Methylphenidate also increases stamina and energy. It has therapeutic effects for major depressive disorders and improves overall mood.

- Modafinil can be used with multiple sclerosis (MS) patients to reduce fatigue. A histamine phosphate/caffeine citrate transdermal patch has also been found to be helpful for MS patients.
- Hydrocortisone used cautiously can enhance mood and improve fatigue for a short time in patients experiencing chronic fatigue syndrome.
- Erythropoietin alpha (epoetin alfa) may treat anemia-based fatigue by working to increase the base hemoglobin levels.
- Antidepressants such as nortriptyline and amitriptyline have shown effectiveness for fatigue.
- CNS stimulants such as dextroamphetamines may be used cautiously.

Nursing measures to help cancer related fatigue

Education is the best tool nurses have for helping patients fight fatigue. Explanations are important to relate fatigue to the disease process, nutrition, treatments, or the presence of infection and fever that can increase the body's demand for rest. Changes in routine and schedule and increased worry and anxiety can increase fatigue. The patient should be prepared for all procedures, activities, and routines to help reduce energy demands. The nurse can also reduce disruptions to the sleep cycle by establishing routines for bedtime and awakening and providing the longest sleep and rest times possible. Encourage foods that will help maintain energy levels, such as protein, with minimal energy output to eat and digest the foods. Small, frequent meals are suggested.
Careful nursing assessments should note and treat any other symptoms, such as pain, depression, nausea, and vomiting, which may be interfering with the patient's ability to rest.
Provide activities that the patient deems distracting and restorative, such as music, time with nature, or time with family and friends. Help the patient determine what expenditures of energy are most important and which can be removed from their daily lives. Encourage routines including mild exercise, leisure activities, or physical therapy.

Non-pain complaints of patients with terminal illnesses

Patients with cancer often express fatigue and anorexia as the top two reasons for emotional and physical distress. Nausea, constipation, states of delirium or other alterations of mental status, and dyspnea are also frequent. Fatigue encompasses symptoms of tiredness, a lack of energy not related to the amount of rest the patient is getting, diminished mental capacity, and weakness. These symptoms interfere with their ability to perform activities of daily living and are often underdiagnosed or downplayed by the patient as inevitable. Anorexia and cachexia are associated with the general wasting of many terminal illnesses and require careful nutritional management. Nausea and constipation are often related to medications and other treatments but are easily treated if assessed and planned for. Palliative treatments are helpful for altered mental states and dyspnea as well.

Sickle cell disease

Sickle cell disease is one of the most common genetic diseases in the United States, generally affecting those of African, Middle Eastern, Mediterranean, and Indian decent. Sickle cell disease is identified by the signature presence of an abnormal globulin gene that allows hemoglobin S to form a "sickle" shape rather than round. This sickle shape shortens the lifespan of the hemoglobin, causing a chronic anemic state. Pallor, jaundice, weakness, and fatigue are common symptoms. A crisis occurs when the cells clump together, causing thrombi, vascular occlusions, hypoxia, and even myocardial infarction. It is also associated with multiple acute pain events. Pain episodes are individualized and can vary in both frequency and severity. A sickle cell crisis is identified by pale lips, tongue, palms, or nail beds, lethargy and difficulty awakening, listlessness, irritability, severe pain, or high fever for at least 2 days. The sickle cell patient is also at higher risk for bacterial infections. Children with sickle cell disease are generally hospitalized less than 6 times a year. In the patient older than 20 years, more than 3 hospitalizations in a year may be an indication of impending death.

Causes of fever in palliative care patients

Minor complications such as constipation and dehydration can be responsible for fever. In the immunosuppressed patient, fresh fruits and vegetables, spices, flowers, and tobacco can be causative factors. Cancers such as Hodgkin and non-Hodgkin lymphoma, hypernephroma, carcinoma of the liver, leukemia, multiple myeloma, Ewing sarcoma, adrenal carcinoma, and obstructive tumors affecting the thermoregulatory system, gastrointestinal, genitourinary, and respiratory systems can all cause fever. Neutropenia, immunosuppression, chemotherapeutic agents, and blood products may also be responsible. Infections, inflammatory processes (thrombophlebitis, trauma, necrosis, pulmonary embolism, ulcerative colitis), autoimmune (lupus, rheumatoid arthritis, AIDS, medication based) and allergic responses, and environmental agents can also cause fever.

Pneumonia in hospice patients

Pneumonia is the most common infection among palliative and hospice patients. Hospice patients are greatly hindered in their physical activity by their disease processes. Many of these patients have immune systems that are also compromised. These factors make them at high risk to develop pneumonia. *Pneumocystis carinii* pneumonia is a specific and common complication of AIDS. Up to 85% of AIDS patients will develop *Pneumocystis carinii* pneumonia without proper preventative treatment. It can, however, be treated prophylactically. Trimethoprim-sulfamethoxazole (TMP-SMZ) is the first drug of choice. Pneumonia presents with fever, dyspnea, and cough. Vaccination is recommended for palliative care patients.

Neutropenia

Neutropenia is identified as a polymorphonuclear neutrophil count equal to or less than 500/mL. Chronic neutropenia is a sustained condition of minimal neutrophils lasting 3 or more months. Neutropenia may occur from a decreased production of white blood cells (eg, from chemotherapy or radiation therapy). It may also occur from a loss of white blood cells from autoimmune disease processes. Neutropenia is silent but dangerous. It leaves essentially no neutrophils to fight any threat of infection. Neutrophils make up as much as 70% of the white bloods cells circulating in the blood. Neutropenia can be the cause of a septic situation, which can be life-threatening. Up to 70% of patients experiencing a fever while in a neutropenic state will die within 48 hours if not treated aggressively.

Lymphedema

Lymphedema results from untreated or incurable edema. It is a chronic condition marked by swelling and accumulated fluids within the tissue. This accumulation is a result of lymphatic drainage failure, inadequate lymph transport capacity, an increased lymph production, or a combination of these. Primary disease is a result of inadequately developed lymphatic pathways, while the secondary disease process is due to damage outside of the pathways. The process is worsened and complicated as macrophages are released to control inflammation caused by the increased release of fibroblasts and keratinocytes. There is a gradual increase in adipose tissue and leakage of lymph through the skin. The skin and tissues gradually thicken and change in color, texture, tone, and temperature. It begins to blister and produce hyperkeratosis, warts, papillomatosis, and elephantiasis. There is an ever-increasing risk of infection and further complications.

Delirium

Delirium is an acute or subacute, reversible state of confusion. Its time frame for onset is very short, over a period of hours or days, and resolving over days or weeks. The severity of delirium fluctuates with the time of day, becoming worse at night. Thinking is impaired and clouded and can fluctuate rapidly in terms of awareness of the surrounding environment. The patient presents with impaired short-term memory and poor attention span with an inability to focus and sustain attention. The patient is disoriented to time and place. Delusions and hallucinations are common. They are usually fleeting, poorly organized, and commonly become multisensory. Speech often becomes uncharacteristic for the patient. It can be loud and rapid or too slow. Psychomotor activity may be increased or reduced. It becomes unpredictable, a variable depending on the delirium experiences. Sleep cycles are often disturbed and can become reversed.

Factors predisposing the elderly to delirium

Age-related changes within the brain such as atrophy, plaque formation, hippocampus, amygdala, or thalamus disorders, Alzheimer disease, and cerebrovascular disease all contribute to patient delirium. Visual changes and hearing loss can cause confusion. Prolonged immobility, Foley catheters, and intravenous lines can factor into delirium, as well as various infections such as pulmonary and urinary tract infections. Metabolism changes including reduction of protein binding of drugs, enhanced effect of opioids, and a reduced ability to eliminate drugs can cause chemical buildup. This polypharmacy can cause increased side effects such as delirium. Malnutrition resulting in vitamin or folate deficiencies, as well as reduced thirst with fluid and electrolyte imbalances and hypovolemia, can also add complications. Cancer and cardiovascular, pulmonary, renal, hepatic, and endocrine diseases are prone to delirium.

Dementia

Dementia is defined as a progressive, irreversible state of decline in metal function. Dementia is chronic and irreversible. Its onset is quiet and slow. Symptoms do not change over the course of the day. Mental clarity remains intact until the later stages, but may be complicated by delirium. Short-term memory may be affected early on but attention span generally remains intact until later stages. Orientation to person, place, and things remain unaltered until later stages when the person may have difficulty recognizing familiar and common objects (anomia) or recognizing familiar people (agnosia). The patient experiences aphasia, a difficulty finding appropriate words and expressing thoughts clearly. Delusions and hallucinations are most often absent. Psychomotor activity is generally unaffected but the patient may exhibit signs of apraxia, a difficulty initiating purposeful movement. Sleep and wake cycles become fragmented.

Interventions for dementia

Individuals with advanced dementia should have minimal stimulation, with simple and consistent routines. Health care providers should use straightforward communication techniques with uncomplicated words and explanations. Patient safety is a high priority, including well-fitting clothing and footwear and an uncluttered, unchanging environment free from as many hazards as possible, such as dimly lit areas, open flames, sharp corners, and loose area rugs. The patient experiencing dementia requires close supervision and should be discouraged from sleeping during daytime hours to avoid time disorientation and to maximize nighttime restfulness and safety. A limited benefit may be obtained in some patients from treatment with donepezil, tacrine, or gingko biloba. All patients with dementia can benefit from careful medication monitoring for interactions and side effects that could add to the patient's condition.

Nonpharmacological interventions for agitation

Maintaining or creating a calm, familiar environment with restricted stimulation is the most effective nonpharmacological intervention for agitation. Furnishings and decorations should be minimal and soothing in nature. Several attempts should be made to reorient and calm the agitated patient with supportive listening, a composed affect, and a calm, gentle, and respectful tone of voice. The agitated individual should be addressed with respect, explaining all actions and procedures in reassuring tones. Consistent reorientation to the patient's surroundings and well-established routines may also provide a calming effect. Music, offered in soft, soothing tones, can also be helpful. The presence of a calming, familiar, and respected family member can provide for agitation reduction as well.

Haloperidol

Haloperidol is an antipsychotic and antiemetic that blocks postsynaptic dopamine receptors in the brain. It is the most appropriate drug for agitation associated with physical harm by the patient to self or others and/or psychotic tendencies. Haloperidol is also useful for opioid-induced, chemical, and mechanical sources of nausea, especially in the presence of anxiety that is aggravating the symptoms. When used in combination with corticosteroids, it can be helpful for chemotherapy-induced nausea and vomiting. The recommended dosage is 0.5 to 5 mg orally every 6 to 24 hours. Other dosages include 5 mg intramuscularly every 3 to 4 hours; or 0.5 to 2 mg IV every 3 to 4 hours. Elderly patients usually require lower initial doses and a more gradual dosage titration. Common side effects include prolonged and involuntary contraction of muscles, a restricted ability to control muscle movement, or an actual loss of muscle movement. Most side effects are minimized by the use of low doses. Haloperidol may have an additive effect when combined with other CNS depressants.

Chemotherapy use with palliative care patients

Chemotherapy may be offered during palliative care to enhance patient comfort, well-being and symptom control for enhanced quality of life. It is understood that the treatment is not expected to provide a cure and should not be given as a means to maintain a sense of false hope within the patient or family. It should be clear that the expectation of treatment is prolonged survival and control of cancer related symptoms. Not all patients will benefit from palliative chemotherapy. The decision to provide chemotherapy is based on the clinical indicators and the patient's wishes. The benefit and cost ratios of treatment need to be considered. Tumor response to treatment, metastasis, and other disease specific factors will help define chemotherapy's usefulness for an individual patient. Patients also need to be aware that chemotherapy involves a commitment to repeated travel, hospitalizations, invasive procedures and assessments in order to make an informed decision.

Classifications of chemotherapeutic agents

The major chemotherapy agents are alkylating agents, antimetabolites, plant alkaloids, antitumor antibiotics, and steroid hormones.

- Alkylating agents work directly by attacking the DNA of cancers such as chronic leukemias, Hodgkin disease, lymphomas, and lung, breast, prostate, and ovary cancers.
- Nitrosoureas inhibit repair in damaged DNA. They are able to cross the blood-brain barrier and are frequently used to treat brain tumors, lymphomas, multiple myeloma, and malignant melanoma.
- Antimetabolites block cell growth. This class of chemotherapeutic drugs is used to treat leukemias, choriocarcinoma, gastrointestinal, and breast and ovary cancers.
- Antitumor antibiotics are a broad category of agents that bind to DNA and prevent RNA synthesis and are use with a wide variety of cancers.
- Plant (vinca) alkaloids are extracted from plants and block cell division. These are used to treat acute lymphoblastic leukemia, Hodgkin and non-Hodgkin lymphomas, neuroblastomas, Wilms tumor, and lung, breast, and testes cancers.
- Steroid hormones have an unclear action but may be useful in treating hormone-dependent cancers such as ovary and breast cancer.

Major routes of chemotherapy delivery

Chemotherapy treatments may be provided orally, intramuscularly or subcutaneously, intravenously, intra-arterially, intralesionally (directly into the tumor), intraperitoneally, intrathecally, or topically. Oral chemotherapy is the easiest and often used in the home. Intravenous delivery is the most common chemotherapy route but intramuscular delivery may have more lasting effects. The goal of intra-arterial chemotherapy is to introduce the agent directly into the blood supply feeding the tumor or affected organ. Ovarian cancer with tumors greater than 2 centimeters in diameter may be treated with intraperitoneal therapy. Acute lymphocytic leukemia is primarily treated with intrathecal administration. Intralesional treatments are used for melanoma and Kaposi sarcoma. Topical treatment is most common with skin cancers.

Common side effects of chemotherapy

Not every patient will experience every symptom, or in the same degree. Side effects can vary greatly; some can be easily controlled with additional medications. Many side effects are due to the effects of the chemotherapy on cells, such as bone marrow, hair and gastrointestinal cells, which have a rapid mitotic rate and rapid turn over. Common side effect can include bone marrow suppression, hair loss (alopecia), mouth ulcers, sore throat and gums, heartburn, nausea, vomiting, loss of appetite, weight loss, anorexia and cachexia, anemia, nerve and muscle problems, dry or discolored skin, kidney and bladder irritation, fatigue, increased bruising and bleeding and infection. The patient's sexual function can also be affected, including possible infertility.

Risks associated with chemotherapy treatment

Infection is a common concern because of the decreased number of neutrophils in the patient's system. Neutropenia is silent but dangerous, leaving no neutrophils to fight the threat of infections. Neutropenia can cause a septic situation, which can be life-threatening. Severe anemia may result in the need for blood transfusions. Neurological damage may include mild alterations in taste or smell, peripheral neuropathy, mental status changes, or seizures. Some anticancer drugs can cause heart damage if not monitored closely. Many anticancer drugs cause kidney damage, as well as increasing the risk of drug toxicity from decreased renal function. Anticancer drugs can also cause cataracts and retina damage.

Cultural considerations for symptom management

Cultural considerations for symptom management are discussed below:
- American Indian and Alaskan natives may be embarrassed to report nausea, vomiting, constipation, or diarrhea. Dyspnea may be described as "heavy air." The patient may maintain the appearance of high activity levels despite fatigue or declining health. Depression and other psychiatric problems may be identified in vague physical symptoms, such as "heart problems."
- Asian and Pacific Islanders feel many illnesses are caused by problems with their "yin" and "yang" and may try to treat their symptoms homeopathically. Mental difficulties are often hidden and not discussed.
- Black populations are generally willing to discuss their symptoms but may be unwilling to seek sufficient treatments, especially medication.
- Hispanic populations are willing to discuss symptoms but may feel the symptoms are beneficial or do not require treatment. Mental difficulties are also considered a weakness and embarrassment.

Practice Issues

Interdisciplinary team roles

The roles of each person who can participate on the interdisciplinary team are explained below:
- Medical director: Oversees and takes responsibility for all care components of the program.
- Primary care physician: Continues direct medical care of their patient but is not required to make home visits or take responsibility for all components of their care.
- Case manager: Coordinates and oversees the implementation of the care plan as it has been defined by the entire care team.
- Nurse: Responsible for the holistic assessment, physical care, and comfort of the patient, within their scope of practice, as well as patient and family education.
- Home health aide: Provides basic physical and comfort care and assists with all activities of daily living.
- Chaplain/Pastor: Meets the patient and family's spiritual needs with patience, flexibility, and respect for beliefs that are different from their own.
- Social worker/psychosocial: Provide psychosocial, family, social/emotional, grief, and bereavement assessment and interventions as needed.
- Professional/Consultive: Provides unique expertise and perspectives as needed.
- All members work together to establish specific patient plans of care. Other companions and volunteers may be utilized as needed.

Benefits of interdisciplinary teamwork in end-of-life care

In an interdisciplinary team, patient and family needs and preferences are assessed by individual group members from different disciplines with their own knowledge and expertise. Each contributing member is trained to see and meet specific patient and family needs. The goal of interdisciplinary teamwork is to involve the patient and family, as well as all care providers, in all decisions. With this cooperative method, a care plan can be developed that meets the goals identified by all parties. Members of the team blend roles, share information, and work together with the patient and family to define coordinated care goals and provide continuity of care. Utilizing numerous disciplines builds a support community for the family and blends their physical, psychosocial, spiritual, and bereavement needs into a cooperative problem-solving network. Success of the interdisciplinary team lies in its ability to approach patient care both scientifically and holistically.

Possible conflicts in care team dynamics

According to Kane, stress and tension can arise when ethics and goals conflict regarding patient care. Eight problems may occur within a team:
- Overwhelming the patient: The amount of information or individual health care team members that need to be dealt with may be intimidating.
- Patient participation: At times, asking the patient for input and decisions is beyond their abilities while dealing with an illness.
- Suppressing individual team members: Non–health care providers may feel unequal.
- Lack of accountability: Tension can build when team members see things outside of their scope left undone.

- Team process over client outcome: The ultimate goal of client well-being can become lost in team dynamics.
- Orthodoxy and groupthink: The group can become closed to new ideas and input.
- Overemphasis on health and safety goals: Care becomes rote and "by the rules" regardless of patient need.
- Resource allocation: High cost resources pose many types of dilemmas.

Effective conflict negotiation

The following are 5 steps to effective conflict negotiation:
1. Identify the source of the conflict: Identify the surrounding circumstances. What did each party contribute, including emotionally, to the situation? What effects has the conflict created on the participants and surrounding community?
2. Address the conflict: Begin identifying active solutions that can create resolution and achieve the group's original purpose.
3. Identify each individual's purpose: Identify what each member can contribute to the solution. Identify common ground and differences.
4. Explore the conflict further: Listen to each participant's account of the events surrounding the conflict. Process and confirm your impression surrounding each account.
5. Problem solve: Confirm which options will meet the most important concerns and interests of each party. Identify the tasks of each side to reach an accommodation and develop standards, communication, and procedures for dealing with the defined conflict in the future.

Collaborating with the attending physician

Collaboration with the attending physician requires sharing of both knowledge about the patient and responsibility for care. Collaboration begins with good communication, as a mutual relationship of respect is essential. The hospice and palliative care nurse must recognize that physicians may have a different perspective on care and may utilize a different approach to communication. At the onset, the nurse should ask pertinent questions and provide input from the nursing perspective about the patient's needs. The nurse should provide regular updates to the physician about any changes in the patient's condition or patient's needs and should respond promptly to any communications from the physician. The nurse should ask about the physician's office hours and the best times and forms (secure email, telephone, face-to-face) to contact the physician for noncritical issues and critical issues. The nurse should also ask how often the physician would like routine updates. The nurse should be frank and assertive but avoid conflict or assigning blame if problems arise.

Qualifying for admission to hospice services and recertification of hospice services

For admission to hospice services under CMS guidelines, a patient must be terminally ill with a life expectancy of 6 months or less. Verbal or written certification that the patient is terminally ill must be received within 2 days after the beginning of the first and following certification periods and may be received up to 15 days prior to the certification/recertification periods. Written certification (rather than verbal), however, must be received before Medicare can be billed. Initial certification must be signed by both the physician and the hospice medical director. The first two certification periods are for 90 days, but with the third period (beginning on day 180) and subsequent recertification periods, the physician must recertify, based on a face-to-face assessment, that the patient's life expectancy is 6 months or less. Assessments may be completed directly by a

- 68 -

physician or a nurse practitioner who provided the findings of the clinical assessment to the certifying physician.

Appropriate times to refer a patient to hospice

It is appropriate to refer a patient and family to hospice when you notice a sudden or steady decline in the patient's condition. If there is a steady loss of function and prognosis is 1 year or less, or when the patient or family are becoming more insistent with their questions and needs, referral to hospice care is appropriate. Hospice can provide support and answers for both the patient and family to meet their increasing anxiety, as well as help with advance directives and care planning. Other indicators that can gauge the need for a referral are the number of hospitalizations in the past year; more than two can indicate disease progression. Also, the onset of multiple new problems and an increase in unpleasant symptoms are reasons for a hospice evaluation. Hospice can help patients who need more palliative symptom relief even while they pursue any treatment methods they choose.

Institute of Medicine recommendations for improving end-of-life care

The Institute of Medicine has the following health care improvements regarding end-of-life care.
- Create and promote reliable, skilled, and supportive care.
- Provide committed health care providers who are informed and dedicated to improving pain and other symptom relief, as well as prevention.
- Improve the health care system through measurable outcome tools for quality improvement, coordinated financial systems, and prescription law reforms.
- Establish medical education that provides the knowledge, skills, and attitudes required to provide quality palliative care.
- Establish palliative care as a combination of expertise, education, and research.
- Continue to pursue ways to meet community needs for those individuals nearing death.

Clinical Practice Guidelines as outlined by the National Consensus for Quality Palliative Care

The Clinical Practice Guidelines for Quality Palliative Care outlined by the National Consensus Project are designed to provide a framework for promoting quality palliative care clinical programs. The main goal is to expand excellence and promote quality, as well as further education and research. The Clinical Practice Guidelines provide standards for clinical practice and care. They do not, however, specify protocol for pain or symptom management. There are now financial incentives for hospice provider participation. Nurses can help promote the efforts of the National Consensus Project by encouraging in-service training programs to promote familiarity with the guidelines, and by participating in ongoing quality improvement activities. Care providers can also critically compare and contrast existing guidelines within their facility with the Clinical Practice Guidelines. Areas of difference should be noted and investigated to promote guideline compliance.

Goals of the National Consensus Project for quality palliative care

The following are 5 goals of the National Consensus Project for quality palliative care:
- Identify definitions, philosophies, and principles concerning palliative care that will be nationally recognized.
- Create clinical practice guidelines for high quality care for both the patient and family.

- Enable clinical practices to grow and improve their resources and performance through structural organization and defined requirements.
- Provide key elements of palliative care that may be used in practices where there is an absence of formal care programs.
- Promote quality recognition, initiatives for growth and certification, and stability for reimbursement and practice measures.

Domains of the National Consensus Project Clinical Practice Guidelines

The domains of the National Consensus Project Clinical Practice Guidelines are explained below:
- Domain 1: Structure and Practice of Care – Care is based on the interdisciplinary team's commitment to comprehensive assessment and care of the patient and family, education and quality improvement, and support of each other as a team.
- Domain 2: Physical – Best practices are employed to address the patient's pain and other symptoms, and educate the patient and family and include them in the plan of care.
- Domain 3: Psychological and Psychiatric – Psychological, psychiatric, grief, and bereavement issues are addressed and managed with high standards using pharmacological, nonpharmacological, support, and counseling treatments as needed.
- Domain 4: Social – Comprehensive care plans will take into account family and social dynamics, interpersonal needs, finances, caregiver availability, and access to health care to promote well-being and ease patient and caregiver burdens.
- Domain 5: Spiritual, Religious, and Existential – Assessing, recognizing, respecting, and supporting spiritual concerns and religious beliefs.
- Domain 6: Cultural – Careful consideration is given to assessing, respecting, and accommodating for culture-specific needs. Resources available reflect cultural diversity and the needs of the community.
- Domain 7: Care of the Patient at the End of Life– Recognition of signs and symptoms of death, making appropriate referrals, and educating the patient and family in an appropriate and sensitive manner.
- Domain 8: Ethics and Law – Demonstrating knowledge of federal and state laws, statutes, and regulations while respecting and implementing patient and family goals and choices in the plan of care.

SUPPORT study findings

SUPPORT: Study to Understand Prognosis and Preferences for Outcomes and Risks of Treatment was funded by the Robert Wood Johnson Foundation and published in the Journal of the American Medical Association in 1995. It revealed the following:
- Many patients are dying in hospitals, alone and suffering from unneeded discomfort and treatments they do not want. These treatments may contribute to the patient's pain and prolong the inevitable dying process.
- Physicians and nurses are still undertrained in end-of-life care.
- The public is beginning to hold the medical society to higher accountability for quality palliative care.
- The definition of family is dynamic and ever changing in terms of considerations for palliative care and support.

- The continuing nursing shortage puts additional strain on nurses working in home health, hospice, and nursing homes.
- Communication and education among the patient, family, and health care providers must be improved.

Advocating for hospice and palliative care

The following are 8 ways in which a nurse can advocate for hospice and palliative care:
- Openly verbalizing the importance of quality terminal care and educating the community about issues surrounding end-of-life care.
- Help create and support palliative care communities and recommend other health care providers and others for membership in palliative care communities.
- Identify and recommend other health care providers and others for membership in palliative care communities.
- Request training in bioethics provided by a qualified ethicist.
- Participate in training and education opportunities.
- Assist in establishing and executing methods for consistent ongoing development and education for committee members.
- Assist in formulating policies regarding treatment issues, education, consultations, and documentation.
- Work with insurance companies to provide support and reimbursement for palliative care services.

Role of nursing research in hospice and palliative care

Nursing research in the areas of hospice and palliative care is still in the infancy stage. Evidence-based research can help with better symptom and pain management and improve the quality of care given during end-of-life. This focus involves all aspects of nursing care before, during, and after the death of a patient. Evidence-based outcomes in nursing research help ensure that the practices and treatments are scientifically based and validated, and that the processes and interventions used by nurses are reliable and effective. Further research is still needed in specialized areas of physical, psycho-spiritual, and social dimensions of end-of-life care.

Barriers to the use of nursing research in palliative care

Most research, with limited research funding, focuses on life issues such as rehabilitation and cure rather than death issues. There are few palliative care advocates and limited promotional and educational support in graduate nursing programs. Relationships between nursing researchers and palliative care groups are also limited. Multiple ethical and other sensitive issues have to be considered. Because of the declining nature of the patient, coupled with late referrals to palliative care, longitudinal outcomes are difficult to define and measure. There are limited research models and instrumentations appropriate for use in this population. Research may also interfere with providing quality care to the dying patient and impede an awareness of the individual patient's needs.

Areas in which nurses can experience burnout

The six areas in which the nurse can experience difficulties with burnout are as follows:
- Workload: Excessive workload in an emotionally draining field can cause exhaustion.
- Control: The nurse may lack control or sufficient authority over resources and decision-making models to feel valued and effective in their work environment.
- Reward: Lack of reward can be financial or related to other benefits that are valued by the individual.
- Community: Social support and continuity with other care providers in the health care team can help avoid feelings of isolation.
- Fairness: Fairness expresses the value and self-worth of the worker as part of a team; mutual respect and equal sharing provide a sense of community.
- Values: Individuals should not feel that their job requires them to compromise their personal values and belief systems. Mismatches may occur between career goals and company missions.

CARES model of stress management and self-care skills

C: Creation of a community. A health care community should jointly shoulder the responsibility for meeting a patient's needs. Team members should be supported throughout daily stresses. A healthy community is more aware of daily stresses and deals with them more appropriately than an individual who feels alone and responsible.
A: Awareness of signs and symptoms. Each team member is aware of the signs and symptoms for depression and burnout and assists with stress management.
R: Reinforcement of the self-care. Relaxation and self-rejuvenation helps each person function more effectively and meet the needs of others.
E: Emphasis on health. Healthy eating habits and regular exercise are key components of daily stress relief.
S: Spiritual awareness. There must also be a recognition of faith and spirit that is meaningful to the individual.

Lifestyle management choices to help palliative care nurses cope with work and stressful situations

The caregiver needs to be able to recognize symptoms of unhealthy stress. Practicing good nutrition, exercising, and meditating help control stress. Establish a spiritual belief system and allow yourself time to grieve losses, both personally and as a member of the care team. Maintain a connection with nature, a sense of humor, and an appreciation for music as therapy. Maintain a healthy balance between work, home, and leisure time, and stay connected with family and friends. Find a confidant who can understand your work-related stresses, be open to new ideas and solutions, and do not be afraid to seek help when it is needed.

Emotional responses of nurses dealing with death and dying

The nurse experiences loss in working with dying patients and their families. Grief is the emotional response to these losses and needs to be expressed in order to facilitate adaptive coping. The nurse may experience feelings of anxiety and grief as well as cumulative loss when he or she is unable to cope effectively with each loss. Ineffective coping mechanisms may include avoidance and emotional distance. Additional stressors may result from circumstances requiring the nurse to either withhold or express personal emotions appropriately and empathize with the patient and family. Losses may be compounded beyond the aspects of the death of a patient. It may include the loss of a close relationship with the patient, losses of professional boundaries, and unmet goals and expectations. The nurse may also experience a compromised personal belief system or assumptions about death that make it difficult to overcome a loss.

Providing palliative care education opportunities for all health care providers

Education among clinical care providers creates awareness of the spectrum of care provided by palliative care services and promotes more referrals of patients that can benefit from these types of services. It also provides the individual caregiver with tools to give competent care in death and dying situations that they may encounter in normal practice. Education places an emphasis on the patient's right to die in the manner of their own choosing whenever possible, giving attention to patient comfort and quality of life in all areas of practice. The World Health Organization (WHO) recommends that all physicians, nurses, social workers, and other health care providers share a commitment to gaining and improving knowledge about death and dying. Education on these matters should also be included in all levels of health care training.

Ethics

Ethics is a branch of philosophy that focuses on the moral life. It is the method used to understand and examine social customs, norms, and rules that help define right and wrong. Ethics are not absolute; they do not have clear answers. They must adjust to cover ever-changing social and cultural contexts and are influenced by individual and cultural morals. Clinical information must incorporate information about the patient and family's values and goals, identification of key decision makers, and consideration of the ethical principles that influence the situation. Nurses should demonstrate a basic understanding of ethical principles and concepts that influence health care and nursing. They also should be knowledgeable about the laws that govern nursing care and the ethical positions of professional nursing organizations. A problem-solving approach, such as the use of the nursing process, should be used to resolve ethical dilemmas. Resolution of ethical dilemmas means that the best choice is made based on all the information considered. Ethical dilemmas can often be resolved without input from the legal system.

Legality and ethics

Laws are guided by societal norms and morals that define the culture's perceptions of right and wrong. Ethics are generally the basis of right and wrong and guide the formation of societal law. However, it is possible to have legal actions that are considered unethical by some groups. For example, assisted suicide, which is legal in Oregon, is considered unethical by many. Other examples include debates over abortion and capital punishment. Conversely, other acts may be illegal but debated as ethical, such as euthanasia. The US Supreme Court determines if a situation or act is constitutional. However, it is still left up to the individual court's interpretation in specific situations.

Euthanasia

Euthanasia is deliberately ending the life of a person with a terminal or incurable chronic illness to end suffering. It is commonly termed "mercy killing." Active euthanasia is defined as knowingly assisting in the death of a patient in order to relieve that patient's suffering. Euthanasia can be further categorized as voluntary (initiated at the request of the terminally ill individual) or involuntary (the decision and request come from a third party when the individual is unable to speak or make decisions). Euthanasia is usually accomplished by the administration of a lethal injection. Currently, euthanasia is illegal in all 50 states and should not be confused with assisted suicide, which is legal in Oregon. Assisted suicide differs from euthanasia in that only the means to end a life are provided. The patient is responsible for actually committing the act of suicide.

Assisted suicide

Assisted suicide is defined as "making a means of suicide available to a patient" (providing pills, chemicals, or weapons) with the prior knowledge of the patient's intention to use the materials to end his or her life. Though the means and method are provided by another individual, the patient is physically capable and mentally competent and ultimately performs the act of suicide. Assisted suicide is the topic of many ethical discussions and legal actions. Another individual must become involved for the patient to commit suicide; the act cannot be committed without assistance. Physician-assisted suicide generally involves the prescription from a physician for a lethal dose of a medication for the patient's use. Physician-assisted suicide is currently only legal in the United States in Oregon, where it became legal in 1997.

Nonmaleficence

Hippocrates was the founder of the principle of nonmaleficence. He advised his students of the principle, *primum non nocere*, which means "First, do no harm." Nonmaleficence is the obligation of the health care provider to avoid exposing the patient to anything unnecessary, risky, or harmful. This ethical principle often comes into play when determining treatments for the patient. It calls into question whether a specific treatment may cause additional suffering without maintaining or increasing the patient's desired quality of life. Nonmaleficence also involves the principle of informed consent, which assumes the patient and family are included in the analysis of purposes for treatment and their results, whether positive or harmful.

Virtue ethics, deontological ethics, and consequentialism

Virtue ethics is the Greek philosophy of character attributes necessary to live a good life. These include courage, loyalty, and civic friendship. These virtues are developed through training and role modeling with virtuous individuals.
Deontological ethics focuses on the rules and motives for behaviors. The morality of an action is based on following rules; it is an obligation of society to act in a virtuous manner. This branch of ethics encompasses the principles of both nonmaleficence and beneficence.
Consequentialism is based on the direct relationship between an action and its consequences. Consequentialists argue that decisions of action should be based directly on the possible and desired outcomes of the action. Individual rights are sometimes sacrificed in favor of the "greater good."

Conscientious objection

Conscientious objection supports the right of persons to refuse to participate in acts that they deem unethical. This can encompass medical treatments or the withholding thereof. It is widely accepted in health care practice, working in the favor of both the patient and provider. It allows patients to accept or refuse treatments based on their religious, ethical, or moral background. It also allows clinicians who are morally opposed to acts such as abortion, capital punishment, and assisted suicide to refrain from caring for patients based on their personal religious, ethical, or moral grounds. No special permission from a governing board is required to act as a conscientious objector; however, nurses must ensure that the patient is not abandoned and his or her wishes are still legally honored. It should be noted that a lack of knowledge regarding the situation is not considered an acceptable reason to object to caring for a patient based on conscientious objection.

Informed consent

Informed consent is a legal procedure to be sure that an individual has the knowledge to give permission for an act to be performed. This knowledge is dependent on the person understanding the facts and implications associated with that act. Informed consent requires the person to be in a position to exercise his or her choice. The individual must be free from any state that could impair their judgment at the time of consent. The health care provider is obligated to provide full disclosure of information regarding the material risks, benefits of the proposed treatment, alternatives, and consequences of no treatment, so that the patient can make an informed choice.

Confidentiality

Confidentiality is a basic patient right of privacy regarding personal and medical matters. Patients must be sure in the knowledge that they may safely discuss any matter with their health care provider in the interest of receiving the best care possible, including a successful, caring, and effective diagnosis and treatment. Privacy must be maintained by keeping confidences and not sharing or discussing any patient information with a third party not privileged to this knowledge. Knowledge by a third party must also never be assumed and permission must be obtained from the patient for discussion in extenuating circumstances. The only time this confidentiality is overruled is when it involves a clear and evident threat to the health or well-being of another individual. Cases of public health concern must also be reported through proper channels and procedures without compromising the patient's privacy. In such cases, it becomes illegal and unethical to withhold pertinent information.

Promoting Excellence programs

The Robert Wood Johnson Foundation created the Promoting Excellence in End-of-Life Care program in 1997 as grant opportunities for those reaching for excellence in family-centered palliative care. The goal is to identify populations that are underserved by palliative care and create gold-standard programs in those areas. Promoting Excellence offers valuable information on how to approach current problems from new angles and provide research outlets for better outcomes, leading to strong, successful, and sustainable programs for all palliative care patients. Areas of concern are feasibility, acceptability, sustainability, quality, and financial ramifications regarding palliative care options. Some of these models focus on providing care in disease-based programs; others focus on the involvement of the family and volunteers in patient care. Education is a key focal point of the program.

Nursing competencies outlined in the report Peaceful Death

The following are the 15 nursing competencies outlined in the report Peaceful Death:
- Recognize dynamic changes in demographics, health care economics, and service delivery that require improved end-of-life care.
- Promote providing comfort to the dying patient as a legitimate, important, and desirable nursing skill.
- Promote effective and compassionate communication with the patient and family.

- Come to terms with their own values, attitudes, and feelings related to death, and accept the diversity of beliefs in others.
- Show respect for the patient and his or her wishes.
- Collaborate with interdisciplinary teams.
- Use standardized assessment tools.
- Plan for and provide care that combines new knowledge with traditional and complimentary management.
- Evaluate patient outcomes effectively.
- Assess and treat the patient holistically.
- Support the patient, family, and friends through their suffering, grief, and bereavement.
- Apply legal and ethical principles to difficult end-of-life issues.
- Promote the effective use of resources.
- Implement quality care in a changing and complex health care environment.
- Continue to obtain and apply new knowledge to improve the quality of care.

Future trends predicted for healthcare delivery in the next twenty years

The number of people with Alzheimer disease may increase from 4 million to 14 million by 2050. The nursing shortage will likely continue, placing particular strain on those in the community health sector. The current life expectancy is not expected to change in the next 20 years. Nursing roles in hospice and palliative care will likely expand to include providing skilled assessment, supportive interventions, consumer education, care coordination, and program leadership. Providers will need to expand their training in caring for younger people with HIV/AIDS and for an increasing number of older people with chronic diseases. Greater emphasis will continue to be placed on resource allocation and research for quality, cost-effective care.

Practice Test

Practice Questions

1. A 67-year-old terminally ill patient wishes to receive comfort care measures in his home. The patient's physician recommends placement in a hospice facility so that Medicare will cover the cost of hospice care. Which of the following statements most accurately describes the Medicare hospice benefit?
   a. The Medicare hospice benefit applies to patients who have a life expectancy of 12 months or less.
   b. The Medicare hospice benefit does not cover the cost of medications used to treat symptoms of terminal illness.
   c. The Medicare hospice benefit covers the cost of hospice services in multiple settings, including the patient's home.
   d. Services provided under the Medicare hospice benefit vary from state to state.

2. A 24-year-old palliative care patient with terminal osteosarcoma takes oral narcotics regularly for the treatment of bone pain. Because of a misunderstanding at the pharmacy, his prescription for narcotic medication is filled 48 hours late, and he develops symptoms of opiate withdrawal, which is most consistent with which of the following?
   a. Psychological dependence (ie, addiction) on narcotic medication
   b. Physical dependence on narcotic medication
   c. Tolerance to narcotic medication
   d. Underuse of prescribed narcotic medication

3. The primary goal of palliative sedation, also known as "terminal" or "total" sedation, in the patient with a terminal illness is:
   a. Relief of intractable pain or suffering
   b. Hastening of death
   c. Improved oxygenation
   d. Reduction in opioid medication doses

4. A home hospice patient becomes progressively less mobile and is ultimately bed-bound. A common complication of immobility in the palliative care patient is:
   a. Myoclonus
   b. Pathological fractures
   c. Pressure ulcers
   d. Pruritus

5. Assessment of a palliative care patient's spiritual or religious beliefs should encompass which of the following?
   a. Screening for spiritual beliefs that may conflict with the palliative care nurse's religious practices
   b. Encouraging the patient to join a religious community if they do not already belong to one
   c. Asking about spiritual customs or rituals around illness and death that are meaningful to the patient
   d. Assessing spiritual or religious beliefs only if the patient volunteers information about religion and spirituality

6. After the history, physical examination, and urinalysis, a useful initial tool in assessing urinary incontinence in the palliative care patient is:

    a. Urodynamic testing

    b. A multiday bladder log

    c. Spinal magnetic resonance imaging

    d. A trial of systemic hormone replacement therapy

7. If an adult patient is concerned about the emotional effect of his terminal illness on his 7-year-old child, the hospice nurse should explain that:

    a. A 7-year-old child is not old enough to understand serious illness and death

    b. Changing family routines will help the child come to terms with the illness

    c. There are age-appropriate ways to assist a child through the grieving process

    d. It is helpful to let the child overhear other family members talking about the death of the parent rather than having a direct conversation

8. A benefit of using a pain assessment tool (e.g., pain scale) in the palliative care patient is the ability to:

    a. Observe a trend in the patient's response to analgesic therapy

    b. Treat the adverse effects of pain medications

    c. Detect symptoms of drug withdrawal

    d. Differentiate true pain from drug-seeking behavior

9. Patients with AIDS most commonly die as a result of:

    a. Malignancy

    b. Heart failure

    c. Opportunistic infections

    d. Renal failure

10. A terminally ill patient is showing decreased awareness of his surroundings, decreased oral intake of solids or liquids, and is no longer able to get out of bed. The most likely explanation for this constellation of findings is:

    a. Loss of hope

    b. Impending death

    c. Depression

    d. Urinary Retention

11. A 51-year-old hospice patient with metastatic breast cancer is experiencing severe pain in association with daily dressing changes of an ulcerating malignant skin wound. These pain episodes are consistent with:

    a. End-of-dose failure

    b. Spontaneous pain

    c. Incident pain

    d. Psychic pain

12. A 57-year-old patient with end-stage heart failure expresses sadness that she can no longer volunteer in church because of the progression of her disease. The hospice nurse should do which of the following?
   a. Remind the patient that it is not helpful to dwell on how her disease has limited her life.
   b. Advise placement in an outpatient hospice facility given the progression of the heart disease.
   c. Assist the patient in identifying other ways of staying involved with her church.
   d. Remind the patient that things could be much worse.

13. The palliative care advanced practice nurse should be proficient in all of the following EXCEPT:
   a. Providing consultation to other medical professionals in complicated palliative care cases
   b. Providing direct education to patients and caregivers
   c. Administering medication with the primary purpose of hastening death
   d. Maintaining knowledge of current evidence-based evaluation and treatments in palliative care

14. Typical features of late-stage dementia include all of the following EXCEPT:
   a. Urinary retention
   b. Swallowing difficulty
   c. Inability to walk
   d. Incontinence

15. A 62-year-old hospice patient with lung cancer develops shortness of breath and facial swelling. The hospice nurse notes distended neck veins. The most likely explanation for these findings is:
   a. Pleural effusion
   b. Lymphedema
   c. Superior vena cava obstruction
   d. Hypercalcemia

16. Disagreement between family members about the plan of care when a palliative care patient lacks the capacity to make treatment decisions should be managed by:
   a. Pursuing legal action to expedite designation of a single family member as medical decision maker
   b. Encouraging the family to consider and discuss what they believe the patient would choose if he or she were able to express his or her wishes
   c. Informing the family that palliative care planning is inappropriate unless the family can reach an agreement
   d. Encouraging each family member to consider what they would choose for themselves in similar circumstances

17. A 24-year-old hospice patient with terminal leukemia expresses his preference to avoid artificial hydration once he is no longer able to take fluids by mouth. The hospice nurse should explain that:
   a. Artificial hydration can be withheld in accordance with the patient's wishes.
   b. Artificial hydration must be provided because it is unethical to deny a patient basic nutrition and hydration.
   c. Dehydration typically contributes to increased respiratory secretions and vomiting during the dying process.
   d. Without artificial hydration, the patient will likely experience more pain during the dying process.

18. The hospice nurse notices that a 54-year-old palliative care patient with laryngeal cancer is taking unusually frequent sips of oral fluids throughout the day. When asked about it, the patient reports that he is trying to relieve a feeling of dry mouth. Additional therapy for relief of dry mouth that the nurse may recommend to this patient is:
    a. A topical anesthetic rinse
    b. Supplemental oxygen therapy
    c. Mouth breathing
    d. Saliva substitutes

19. A 47-year-old patient with metastatic melanoma receiving opioid analgesic medication informs the hospice nurse that she would "rather just be in pain than feel so sleepy from the pain meds." Given this patient's concerns, the hospice nurse should recommend:
    a. Increased fluid intake and daily stool softeners
    b. The addition of a benzodiazepine to help the patient feel less anxious
    c. Administration of naloxone before each dose of pain medication
    d. Consideration of a psychostimulant medication

20. Common barriers to providing optimal palliative care to patients living in poverty include all of the following EXCEPT:
    a. Fragile or nonexistent housing
    b. Less stable support systems
    c. Undependable transportation to medical visits
    d. Less effective coping skills

21. Patients describing neuropathic pain will most likely characterize their pain as:
    a. Achy, throbbing, and dull
    b. Burning, "pins and needles," and shooting
    c. Pressure, squeezing, and crampy
    d. Diffuse

22. A 39-year-old patient with testicular cancer has progressive disease despite aggressive cancer treatment. He consents to hospice care and is able to articulate his priorities and goals for treatment but continues to state that he is confident he will survive this illness. The patient's wife asks the hospice nurse how to force the patient to "face the truth." The most appropriate response to the patient's wife is:
    a. "He will acknowledge the severity of his illness when he is ready."
    b. "You should just remind him regularly that he will not survive this illness."
    c. "There is always a possibility of a miracle cure."
    d. "You should point out to him all of the things he can no longer do because of his illness."

23. All of the following features of delirium would be expected in the patient with dementia EXCEPT:
    a. Disturbed sleep
    b. Labile mood
    c. Rapid onset
    d. Impaired short-term memory

24. Under the Medicare hospice benefit, respite care for relief of the patient's family caregiver refers to:
    a. Inpatient hospice care for up to 5 consecutive days
    b. Home hospice care for up to 5 consecutive days
    c. Inpatient hospice care for up to 10 consecutive days
    d. Initiation of a "do not resuscitate" order

25. A 43-year-old palliative care patient with amyotrophic lateral sclerosis (ALS) has progressive weakness of the respiratory muscles and complains of dyspnea. Which of the following statements most accurately describes the use of noninvasive positive airway pressure ventilation (eg, BiPAP) in patients with ALS?
    a. BiPAP is not clinically indicated when respiratory insufficiency is due to muscle weakness.
    b. BiPAP in the patient with ALS can lead to prolonged survival and improved quality of life.
    c. Patients with ALS using BiPAP must be in an inpatient setting.
    d. The use of opioid medications for dyspnea is contraindicated in patients using BiPAP.

26. The malignancy most commonly associated with upper extremity lymphedema is:
    a. Prostate cancer
    b. Melanoma
    c. Breast cancer
    d. Brain cancer

27. Fentanyl is administered transdermally (ie, fentanyl patch) to a home hospice patient for treatment of cancer-related pain. Which of the following statements most accurately describes the use of transdermal fentanyl in the palliative care setting?
    a. Transdermal fentanyl administration is helpful for treating pain in the palliative care patient who develops dysphagia.
    b. Heat applied directly over the patch will slow the rate of fentanyl absorption.
    c. Steady-state levels of serum fentanyl are reached within 6 hours of patch application.
    d. Transdermal fentanyl administration is helpful for treating breakthrough pain in the palliative care patient.

28. If a terminally ill 41-year-old patient is concerned that designating a health care power of attorney (ie, proxy) in an advance directive will result in loss of control over end-of-life decisions, the hospice nurse should explain that the:
    a. Designated proxy will only dictate end-of-life decision making if the patient is unable to express his or her wishes.
    b. Patient should only complete an advance directive once he or she is willing to relinquish control of decision making to the designated proxy.
    c. Advance directive is more important with an elderly palliative care patient.
    d. Patient should designate his or her primary physician as the health care power of attorney.

29. A 44-year-old hospice patient has a malodorous malignant wound, which is debrided and cleaned regularly. The hospice nurse can recommend which of the following additional therapies to decrease wound odor?
    a. Topical steroid application
    b. Topical metronidazole application
    c. Systemic metronidazole administration
    d. Calcium alginate dressings

30. Impaired coping by the caregivers of a palliative care patient is most likely expressed as:
    a. Uncertainty and fear
    b. Hope for the future
    c. Resentment about the large amount of attention being paid to the patient
    d. Seeking support resources beyond the palliative care plan

31. Which of the following would most likely lead to inadequate treatment of pain in the palliative care patient?
    a. Mutual trust between provider and patient
    b. Frequent multidimensional pain assessments
    c. Patient concern for developing an addiction to pain medication
    d. Availability of a variety of pain assessment tools

32. According to the American Nurses Association's position statement, a patient's request to not receive artificial hydration or nutrition in association with end-of-life care may be:
    a. Inconsistent with the primary ethical and professional expectations of a palliative care nurse
    b. Decided on an individual case basis and may be consistent with appropriate end-of-life care
    c. Considered a form of active euthanasia
    d. Usually causes discomfort for the terminally ill patient

33. The most effective support system for assisting the hospice nurse in coping with the emotional strain of caring for dying patients and their families is:
    a. A combination of professional and personal support strategies
    b. A change to a different nursing specialty if the nurse is having difficulty coping
    c. A leave of absence to pursue individual stress management treatment
    d. Urging the hospice nurse to deal with his or her grief reactions outside of work

34. Contributors to constipation in the palliative care patient include all of the following EXCEPT:
    a. *Clostridium difficile* infection
    b. Decreased fluid intake
    c. Opioid medications
    d. Hypercalcemia

35. Tricyclic antidepressants are most likely to be effective in treating which of the following types of pain?
    a. Ischemic pain
    b. Cancer-related bone pain
    c. Visceral pain
    d. Neuropathic pain

36. Extensive patient and caregiver participation in interdisciplinary team discussions is important so that the:
    a. Patient and caregivers can be informed of the plan of care as formulated by the medical providers
    b. Cost of hospice care is reimbursed by the patient's insurance provider
    c. Plan of care can be crafted to meet the specific needs and goals of the individual patient and family
    d. Patient and caregivers come to terms with a terminal prognosis

37. Malignant bowel obstruction would most likely develop in a patient with which of the following cancers?
   a. Lung
   b. Breast
   c. Leukemia
   d. Ovarian

38. A 51-year-old patient with terminal breast cancer asks the palliative care nurse if she should try acupuncture for intractable vomiting. The nurse's best response to this patient should be:
   a. "You will need to stop all of your antinausea medications if you choose to pursue acupuncture."
   b. "Acupuncture cannot treat vomiting."
   c. "Some patients find acupuncture a helpful additional therapy for vomiting."
   d. "Alternative medicine is not a proven science."

39. A patient with end-stage chronic obstructive pulmonary disease is dyspneic despite upright positioning and supplemental oxygen administration. The first-line pharmacologic therapy of choice for treating dyspnea in this clinical scenario is:
   a. Benzodiazepines
   b. Glycopyrrolate
   c. Scopolamine
   d. Opioids

40. A 43-year-old patient with ovarian cancer describes a constant, throbbing pain in her lower abdomen for the last 18 hours, which ranges from an intensity of 4 (on a 10-point scale) at rest to 8 with movement. This information best describes which type of pain assessment?
   a. Physiologic and sensory pain assessment
   b. Affective pain assessment
   c. Comprehensive pain assessment
   d. Sociocultural pain assessment

41. A 27-year-old patient with metastatic cervical cancer is receiving 10 mg of morphine per dose intravenously (IV) for cancer-related pain. Because of the side effects associated with morphine, the palliative care team decides to change the patient's IV pain medication from morphine to hydromorphone. The approximate hydromorphone analgesic dosage that is equivalent to a morphine 10 mg IV dose is:
   a. Hydromorphone 15 mg IV
   b. Hydromorphone 1.5 mg IV
   c. Hydromorphone 10 mg IV
   d. Hydromorphone 0.15 mg IV

42. Under the Medicare hospice benefit, general inpatient hospice care would be most appropriate for which of the following patients?
   a. A 64-year-old patient with esophageal cancer who is receiving artificial nutrition through a feeding tube
   b. A 12-year-old patient with leukemia and intractable pain
   c. A 37-year-old patient with AIDS who would like to start a new antiretroviral medication
   d. A 59-year-old patient with congestive heart failure who develops dyspnea

43. The palliative care nurse demonstrates turning maneuvers for pressure ulcer prevention to a patient's family member after describing the factors that contribute to ulcer development. After completion of verbal teaching and demonstration by the nurse, the caregiver should be asked to:
    a. Complete a written examination about turning maneuvers
    b. Practice turning maneuvers, using the nurse as the "patient"
    c. Sign a document, relieving the palliative care team of liability if the patient develops pressure ulcers
    d. Demonstrate the turning maneuvers with the nurse present

44. Therapeutic touch is most accurately described as:
    a. Stimulation of reflex points on the hands and feet, corresponding to body parts
    b. The use of touch while directing healing energy to the patient
    c. The use of essential oils for the purpose of treating inflammation and infection
    d. Body poses with deep breathing to facilitate relaxation and healing

45. A hospice patient is taking amitriptyline for neuropathic pain. Which of the following is an adverse effect of amitriptyline?
    a. Hypersalivation
    b. Weight loss
    c. Diarrhea
    d. Cardiac arrhythmias

46. Diuretic medication (eg, furosemide) for a palliative care patient with severe heart failure would be most helpful for managing which of the following symptoms?
    a. Depression
    b. Chest pain
    c. Dyspnea
    d. Constipation

47. All of the following are components of normal grieving EXCEPT:
    a. Fear
    b. A mix of good and bad days
    c. Anger
    d. Hopelessness

48. Which of the following medications most commonly causes myoclonus in the palliative care patient?
    a. Benzodiazepines
    b. Opioids
    c. Antispasmodics
    d. Antibiotics

49. A 34-year-old hospice patient with metastatic melanoma develops loud, moist-sounding breathing also known as a "death rattle." Which of the following statements most accurately describes the "death rattle"?
    a. The "death rattle" is usually associated with significant patient anxiety.
    b. Suctioning of oral secretions is the first-line treatment of choice for the "death rattle."
    c. Family members are not usually distressed by the patient's "death rattle."
    d. The "death rattle" usually indicates impending death.

50. Bisphosphonates (eg, pamidronate) are most commonly used in the palliative care patient to treat which of the following conditions?
  a. Syndrome of inappropriate diuretic hormone secretion
  b. Hypercalcemia
  c. Cushing syndrome
  d. Hyperglycemia

51. A patient with fourth-stage pancreatic cancer is severely malnourished and barely eating because she has a very bad bitter taste in her mouth all of the time, making food revolting and causing nausea. All of the following strategies may be helpful EXCEPT
  a. Rinse the mouth with a salt and soda solution before eating.
  b. Use a straw to drink liquids.
  c. Eat cold foods and liquids.
  d. Eat highly spiced foods.

52. A patient taking high doses of opioids has had persistent constipation but complains of a sudden episode of diarrhea and increasing urinary incontinence. The most likely cause is
  a. Enteritis.
  b. Fecal impaction.
  c. Allergic response to medication.
  d. Malabsorption syndrome.

53. Which type of pain most often requires opioids to control it?
  a. Visceral.
  b. Neuropathic.
  c. Somatic.
  d. Psychological.

54. A daughter caring for her dying mother expresses frustration with the constant demands of care, stating, "It will be a relief when she dies." The best initial response is
  a. "I'm sure you don't mean that."
  b. "I know your mother appreciates what you are doing for her."
  c. "Caregiving is very difficult and exhausting."
  d. "Why do you say that?"

55. A patient with end-stage renal disease is too confused to make decisions and is still receiving dialysis. Which is the best approach to use to initiate discussion about discontinuing dialysis with family members?
  a. "Do you want to continue dialysis?"
  b. "There is nothing more we can do to help your mother."
  c. "Do you want to stop dialysis and let your mother die?"
  d. "We have exhausted all remedies, and the dialysis is prolonging your mother's suffering."

56. An organ procurement organization is required by federal law to ask family decision makers about organ donation in the absence of an advance directive under what condition?
  a. The patient's death is expected.
  b. The patient dies in the hospital.
  c. The patient dies at home.
  d. Under all circumstances when a patient dies.

57. The cracker test is used to assess for
    a. Nausea.
    b. Candida.
    c. Reflux.
    d. Xerostomia.

58. A daughter expresses fear about dealing with her father's dying at home. What is the best response?
    a. "You can call hospice and a nurse will come to be with you during your father's death."
    b. "I'm sure you will be fine."
    c. "Let's talk about what to expect and what to do."
    d. "You can always transfer your father to the hospital when death is imminent."

59. All of the following medications are usually continued during the final days of life EXCEPT
    a. Antipyretics.
    b. Antihypertensives.
    c. Antiemetics.
    d. Anticonvulsants.

60. A patient with a glioblastoma nearing death has been receiving oral corticosteroids to control cerebral edema but wishes to discontinue the steroids. What is the best approach?
    a. Discontinue the medication without tapering.
    b. Discontinue the medication after tapering.
    c. Discontinue the medication after tapering and increase analgesia.
    d. Discontinue the medication after tapering and increase anticonvulsant and analgesia if necessary.

61. Which of the following is an indication that death may occur in a few hours for a patient with severe cardiorespiratory disease?
    a. Heart rate doubles.
    b. Radial pulse is no longer palpable.
    c. Mottling of extremities is evident.
    d. Nail beds are cyanotic.

62. Anticholinergic drugs may be indicated in the final days of life for treatment of
    a. Nausea.
    b. Cheyne-Stokes respirations.
    c. Death rattle
    d. Agonal respirations.

63. Palliative care should be provided to patients with life-threatening diseases
    a. Throughout the disease process and continuum of care.
    b. Concurrently with curative treatments.
    c. Concurrently with supportive treatment only.
    d. When the patient is referred to hospice care.

64. An 80-year-old woman is caring for her elderly husband who wishes to die at home and is under Medicare home health hospice care. The caregiver appears exhausted and weepy. The best initial solution is
  a. Place patient in a long-term care facility.
  b. Tell caregiver to hire an assistant.
  c. Make daily nursing visits.
  d. Provide in-patient respite care for 5 days.

65. According to Centers for Medicare & Medicaid Services (CMS) regulations regarding the Medicare Hospice Benefit, an interdisciplinary team must include all of the following EXCEPT
  a. Physician.
  b. Nurse.
  c. Nutritionist.
  d. Social worker.

66. According to Byock and Merriman's end-of-life construct, which dimension includes patients' emotions as they near death, including anxiety, fear, readiness, and acceptance?
  a. Physical.
  b. Transcendent.
  c. Interpersonal.
  d. Well-being.

67. One of the developmental landmarks for life completion/closure is accepting the finality of life. One of the tasks associated with this landmark is
  a. Emotional withdrawal.
  b. Accepting new personal definition of self.
  c. Life review.
  d. Self-forgiveness.

68. From a caregiver's perspective, all of the following indicate that the caregiver has accepted the finality of life EXCEPT
  a. Expressing anticipatory grief.
  b. Listening to the patient's life review.
  c. Telling the patient it is all right to die.
  d. Discussing personal loss.

69. According to Harper's stages of adaptation for hospice nurses, a nurse who overidentifies with the patient's situation is in which stage of adaptation?
  a. Stage I, intellectualism.
  b. Stage II, emotional survival.
  c. Stage III, depression.
  d. Stage IV, emotional arrival.

70. A patient recently diagnosed with stage 4 ovarian cancer goes into a rage when having blood drawn, accusing the laboratory technician of purposefully hurting her and demanding that the technician be reprimanded or fired. The best response is
  a. "It can be painful when blood is drawn."
  b. "It's not the laboratory technician's fault."
  c. "I'm so sorry you had to experience discomfort."
  d. "You are absolutely right. We will deal with the technician."

71. When differentiating normal grief processes from depression, all of the following are normal responses to grief and terminal disease EXCEPT:
    a. Patient cries periodically.
    b. Patient does not cry at all.
    c. Patient openly expresses anger.
    d. Patient complains of lack of energy.

72. A caregiver is persistently in denial about her husband's impending death, saying repeatedly, "He just needs to rest, and he'll be ok." What is the best response?
    a. "Your husband is going to die soon."
    b. "It must be very difficult to believe what is happening to your husband."
    c. "What do you think is going to happen?"
    d. "Do you really believe that?"

73. In a state that does not allow physician-assisted death, a patient asks the nurse to assist him in committing suicide. The best initial response of the nurse is
    a. "Assisted suicide is illegal."
    b. "That would be terrible for your family."
    c. "I'm sorry. I can't help you."
    d. "Tell me why you feel you want to die now."

74. According to Piaget's theory of cognitive development, at what age is a child likely to believe that he is the reason his parent is dying?
    a. Age 2 to 7.
    b. Age 7 to 11.
    c. Age 11 to 13.
    d. Age 13 to 15.

75. A family member has called to say that a home hospice patient has died, and to request a nurse come to make the death pronouncement. The first thing the nurse should do when entering the home 20 minutes later is
    a. Check the patient for heart and breath sounds.
    b. Introduce herself to the family.
    c. Look at the patient and confirm death.
    d. Express condolences.

76. A patient who has gone through months of treatment but suffered a relapse is severely depressed and withdrawn. She states, "There's no point to any of this anymore. I want it to be over." Which is the best response?
    a. "Don't give up hope."
    b. "I can see you are depressed, and I'm worried about you."
    c. "Have you considered clinical trials?"
    d. "Have you been thinking of ways of hurting yourself?

77. All of the following are risk factors for complicated bereavement EXCEPT
    a. History of substance abuse.
    b. Recent loss of another family member.
    c. Religious faith.
    d. Loss of income.

78. A woman in the final weeks of life tells the nurse that she feels she has been a failure as a mother. How can the nurse respond to encourage life review?
   a. "What would you do differently?"
   b. "What positive memory do you have of raising your children?"
   c. "I'm sure you did the best you could?"
   d. "That's not important now."

79. All of the following are indications that a patient's drugs are being diverted in the home EXCEPT
   a. The caregiver is increasingly isolating the patient and refusing home care.
   b. The patient has had an abrupt, marked increase of pain.
   c. The patient's pain pills are a different color.
   d. The caregiver is unconventional in appearance.

80. Which of the following religions views embalming as desecration of the body?
   a. Islam.
   b. Hinduism.
   c. Buddhism.
   d. Shintoism.

81. A patient with cancer has poorly controlled pain because she forgets to take her hydrocodone and acetaminophen 5/325 mg tablets on schedule but takes one or two tablets every 3 to 6 hours depending on how severe her pain is. The best solution is probably to
   a. Educate the patient about the importance of staying on schedule.
   b. Switch to fentanyl patch.
   c. Switch to a higher dose of hydrocodone.
   d. Set up an alarm system to remind the patient when the medication is due.

82. Which type of pain assessment is most indicated for a patient whose pain medication dosage has been increased to better control pain?
   a. Comprehensive pain assessment.
   b. Assessment of aggravating factors.
   c. Assessment of location and duration of pain.
   d. Assessment of intensity of pain with 0 to 10 scale.

83. The 5 key elements of pain assessment include words, intensity, location, duration, and
   a. Aggravating/Alleviating factors.
   b. Affect.
   c. Behavior.
   d. Response.

84. Poorly localized pain that is described as cramping, distention, deep, and pressure is most likely
   a. Visceral.
   b. Neuropathic,
   c. Somatic.
   d. Psychological.

85. A patient tells the nurse and doctor that she is barely having any pain and rarely takes pain medications, but her pain medication record shows she has been averaging about 20 to 25 mg of hydrocodone daily. This probably indicates
    a. The patient is actively lying.
    b. The patient is reluctant to admit the degree of pain.
    c. The patient is giving the medication to someone else.
    d. The patient is confused.

86. An older patient with cancer is in much pain and is willing to take other opioids but refuses to take morphine. The probable reason is that the patient
    a. Associates morphine with dying.
    b. Wants stronger medications.
    c. Is confused.
    d. Is afraid of becoming addicted.

87. Which pain scale is most appropriate for use with a 5-year-old child?
    a. CRIES.
    b. FACES (Wong-Baker).
    c. 0-10 pain intensity scale.
    d. CHEOPS.

88. The most appropriate music therapy to aid in relaxation and pain control is
    a. Classical music.
    b. Patient's preference.
    c. Jazz.
    d. New Age.

89. Which of the following medications is appropriate for use as terminal/palliative sedation?
    a. Haloperidol 0.5 to 5 mg every 4 to 12 hours.
    b. Olanzapine 2.5 mg twice daily.
    c. Lorazepam 0.5 to 2 mg every 1 to 4 hours.
    d. Midazolam 0.5 to 6 mg per hour intravenously.

90. A patient receiving morphine experiences severe respiratory depression. Which medication is indicated to control symptoms?
    a. Flumazenil.
    b. N-acetylcysteine.
    c. Neostigmine.
    d. Naloxone.

91. An elderly patient has chemotherapy-induced nausea and vomiting. Which of the following antiemetic agents is most likely to be effective?
    a. Haloperidol.
    b. Scopolamine.
    c. Ondansetron.
    d. Dronabinol.

92. Which of the following adjuvant analgesics is most indicated to relieve pain associated with spinal cord compression?
   a. Pamidronate.
   b. Clonazepam.
   c. Nifedipine.
   d. Prednisone.

93. A palliative care patient is receiving chemotherapy through a port in the upper chest but complains that the needle insertion is very painful, so he becomes very anxious before treatment. Which therapy is most indicated?
   a. EMLA cream.
   b. Extra pain medication.
   c. Relaxation exercises.
   d. Anti-anxiety medication.

94. A patient who is nearing death suffers from refractory pain and is administered ketamine for pain crisis. What other medication adjustments/additions should be made?
   a. Decrease opioid dose by 25%.
   b. Decrease opioid dose by 25% and administer diazepam or lorazepam.
   c. Decrease opioid dose by 50% and administer diazepam or lorazepam.
   d. No adjustments/additions are necessary.

95. A patient who abruptly stops an opioid, after radiotherapy shrinks a tumor, and exhibits withdrawal symptoms has probably developed
   a. Addiction.
   b. Tolerance.
   c. Physical dependence.
   d. Pseudoaddiction.

96. A patient has developed persistent skin irritation from use of fentanyl patches but does not want to change to another medication. What treatment may be used to prevent irritation?
   a. Spray with steroid used for inhalation therapy.
   b. Apply steroid cream.
   c. Apply powder to skin.
   d. Spray with skin barrier.

97. If a patient receives 10 mg of morphine, what is the equianalgesic dose of hydromorphone?
   a. 50 mcg.
   b. 1.5 mg.
   c. 7.5 mg.
   d. 130 mg.

98. Which of the following is an example of a complementary therapy?
   a. Cancer-cure diets.
   b. Oxygen therapy.
   c. Aromatherapy.
   d. Biomagnetic therapy.

99. Which complementary therapy is based on the idea that "like cures like?"
   a. Ayurvedic medicine.
   b. Homeopathy.
   c. Naturopathy.
   d. Traditional Chinese medicine.

100. Based on general cultural differences, which ethnic group tends to be the least expressive when in pain?
   a. Asians.
   b. Hispanics.
   c. Middle Easterners.
   d. Southern European/Mediterranean.

101. A patient is using a 72-hour fentanyl patch to relieve pain and has good pain control for 48 hours but routinely experiences increased pain for the last 24 hours. The best solution is to
   a. Increase the dosage or change the patch more frequently.
   b. Change to a different drug.
   c. Use complementary therapies, such as acupuncture.
   d. Increase the use of oral opioids for the last 24 hours.

102. A patient wants to continue to attend a weekly 1-hour book club meeting, but the meeting is up a flight of stairs and the exertion to climb the stairs results in severe incident pain. What is the best solution?
   a. The patient should stop attending the meeting.
   b. The patient should increase baseline analgesia by 25%.
   c. The patient should take a rapid-onset, short-acting analgesic before the meeting.
   d. The patient should take a long-acting analgesic after the meeting.

103. A patient with end-stage dementia displays an abrupt, aggressive change in behavior. The nurse's initial intervention should be to
   a. Place the patient in a quiet environment.
   b. Evaluate the patient for causes of discomfort.
   c. Administer analgesia.
   d. Administer chemical restraint.

104. Which electrolyte imbalance occurs with syndrome of inappropriate antidiuretic hormone secretion (SIADH)?
   a. Hyponatremia.
   b. Hypernatremia.
   c. Hypocalcemia.
   d. Hypercalcemia.

105. If a patient has just died and the nurse is preparing the body for family arrival, which of the following should the nurse do?
   a. Tie the mouth closed.
   b. Place dentures in the mouth.
   c. Close the eyelids.
   d. Cover the deceased body, including the face, with a sheet.

106. When a patient has received bad news about prognosis, what is the best approach to ascertain the patient's needs?
    a. "Do you need anything to help you cope with this news?"
    b. "I know you have received disappointing news. Can you tell me what I can do to help you?"
    c. "Is everything all right? Can I help you?"
    d. "I feel terrible for you. What can I do?"

107. All of the following are primary benefits of working with an interdisciplinary team EXCEPT
    a. Effective problem-solving.
    b. Pooling of expertise.
    c. Personal support system.
    d. Independent decision-making.

108. When using hypodermoclysis to provide fluids for a patient who is dehydrated, what is the usual initial rate of infusion?
    a. 50 mL/hr.
    b. 100 mL/hr.
    c. 150 mL/hr.
    d. 200 mL/hr.

109. All of the following are effects of dehydration on the pulmonary system at the end of life EXCEPT:
    a. Reduced cough.
    b. Reduced secretions.
    c. Decreased dyspnea.
    d. Increased death rattle.

110. A patient has had a right-hemisphere stroke with left-sided paralysis. Which method of communication is probably indicated?
    a. Speak very slowly, standing on the patient's right side.
    b. Use visual aids, standing on the patient's left side.
    c. Speak normally, standing on the patient's right side.
    d. Use simple vocabulary and gestures, standing on the patient's left side.

111. A patient with Parkinson disease has been evaluated for the ability to swallow, and tests indicate pharyngeal phase dysphagia. Which of the following symptoms should the nurse expect?
    a. Patient chokes while swallowing and often regurgitates food into the nose.
    b. Patient complains of difficulty swallowing but rarely chokes or coughs.
    c. Patient drools, and food remains in the mouth after a meal.
    d. Patient regurgitates food frequently after eating.

112. A patient's records indicate heavy smoking and a history of alcoholism and a diagnosis of variant (Prinzmetal) angina. What type of pain should the nurse anticipate the patient might experience?
    a. Chest pain occurs when the patient is lying flat at rest.
    b. Chest pain occurs cyclically at the same time each day with the patient at rest.
    c. Chest pain occurs after exertion.
    d. Chest pain occurs with increasing frequency after exertion and at rest.

113. Which of the follow triads indicates common risk factors for acute venous thromboembolism?
  a. Virchow's triad.
  b. Beck's triad
  c. Cushing's triad.
  d. Waddell's triad.

114. Microvascular changes in chronic diabetes can lead to all of the following consequences EXCEPT
  a. Blindness.
  b. Diabetic foot ulcer.
  c. Chronic renal failure.
  d. Myocardial infarction.

115. A patient with advanced cirrhosis has marked tense ascites and is experiencing severe dyspnea, pain, and orthopnea. The most appropriate treatment is
  a. Comfort measures only.
  b. Fluid restriction.
  c. Sodium restriction.
  d. Paracentesis.

116. A patient with dysphagia has an order for a mechanically altered diet because of impaired tongue control and limited chewing ability. Which of the following foods is appropriate?
  a. Raw fruit.
  b. Baked fish.
  c. Pureed vegetables.
  d. Soft scrambled eggs.

117. A patient has persistent xerostomia because of postradiation damage to the salivary glands. Which of the following treatment is appropriate to use to stimulate production of saliva?
  a. Bethanechol.
  b. Pilocarpine.
  c. Vitamin C.
  d. Artificial saliva.

118. A patient with gastric cancer and gastric distention has developed chronic hiccoughs, which result in severe pain. Which initial medication is indicated to control the hiccoughs?
  a. Simethicone or metoclopramide.
  b. Baclofen or midazolam.
  c. Gabapentin or carbamazepine.
  d. Haloperidol or chlorpromazine.

119. Which type of laxative is usually most effective for opioid-related constipation in the chronically ill patient?
  a. Saline laxatives.
  b. Osmotic laxatives.
  c. Bulk laxatives.
  d. Stimulant laxatives.

120. The opioid medication that is most likely to cause pruritus is
   a. Oxymorphone.
   b. Fentanyl.
   c. Codeine.
   d. Morphine.

121. Which of the following primary cancers has the highest risk of metastasizing to the bones?
   a. Breast and prostate.
   b. Lung and thyroid.
   c. Pancreas.
   d. Kidney.

122. A patient with an inoperable brain tumor has displacement of cerebral tissue, altered cerebral perfusion, and increased intracranial pressure. What is the best position for the patient?
   a. Flat in bed with head and neck neutral position.
   b. Head of bed raised 10 degrees with head and neck in neutral position.
   c. Head of the bed raised to 30 to 45 degrees with head and neck in neutral position.
   d. Trendelenburg position with head and neck in neutral position.

123. Cancer patients who report severe fatigue and general debility should routinely be assessed for all of the following EXCEPT
   a. Depression.
   b. Sleep disorders.
   c. Anemia.
   d. Family conflict.

124. A patient with ovarian cancer has been losing 2 to 4 pounds weekly because of anorexia/cachexia. All of the following are good strategies to improve intake EXCEPT:
   a. Small frequent meals.
   b. Nutritional drinks, such as Ensure.
   c. Advise patient that she must eat to live.
   d. Explore dietary preferences with patient.

125. A patient with urge incontinence is taking immediate-release oxybutynin to decrease bladder contractility, but complains that the dry mouth it causes makes her very uncomfortable. Which of the following alternative drugs is likely to cause the least mouth dryness?
   a. Extended-release tolterodine.
   b. Propantheline.
   c. Hyoscyamine oral tablets.
   d. Flavoxate.

126. A patient with stage 4 liver cancer is planning to receive care under the Medicare Hospice Benefit. Which of the following services will be covered by this benefit?
   a. Extended live-in 24-hour care.
   b. Ambulance service, arranged for by family member.
   c. Antibiotics to treat a urinary infection.
   d. Service at a private, non–Medicare-approved hospice.

127. A patient under hospice care lives with her son who works outside of the home, so she spends many hours at home alone with her cat. Which of the following volunteer services may provide the most benefit?
    a. Transportation services.
    b. Friendly visitors.
    c. Pet walkers.
    d. Hair stylists.

128. A hospice patient tells the nurse that she has so many questions to ask her doctor but she gets nervous and flustered and forgets what to ask. What is the best response?
    a. "Let's make a list of questions to give to the doctor."
    b. "You should make a list of questions."
    c. "I'll tell the doctor you have questions."
    d. "Perhaps I can answer your questions."

129. A patient has severe lower extremity lymphedema. Which prophylactic treatment is generally recommended?
    a. Corticosteroids.
    b. Antifungal powders.
    c. Antibiotics.
    d. Oral antifungal agents.

130. Which of the following support surfaces for prevention of pressure sores has low moisture retention?
    a. Static water flotation.
    b. Alternating air.
    c. High air loss.
    d. Foam.

131. A hospice patient resists turning and has developed a coccygeal ulcer that appears as a blistered area with a wound bed that is red/pink with slight exudate but without slough and only partial-thickness skin loss (National Pressure Ulcer Advisory Panel [NPUAP] stage II). The best dressing choice is
    a. Semi-permeable film.
    b. Hydrocolloid.
    c. Alginate.
    d. Gauze.

132. A patient has Medicare and supplementary insurance but is concerned about direct nonmedical costs, which include
    a. Durable medical equipment.
    b. Physician's visits.
    c. Lost income from employment.
    d. Emergency services.

133. A patient with breast cancer has complained of increasing fatigue and dyspnea and has developed a dry, nonproductive cough with dull pain in the left chest. The left lung field is dull to percussion with decreased breath sounds and decreased diaphragmatic excursion. The most likely cause is
    a. Lung metastasis.
    b. Pulmonary embolism.
    c. Pleural effusion.
    d. Pneumothorax.

134. Which of the following is likely to have the most negative impact on a patient's ability to maintain a feeling of hope at the end of life?
    a. Pain is poorly controlled.
    b. Patient lives alone.
    c. Patient has no religious faith.
    d. Patient has signed a DNR request.

135. The gay partner of a closeted man who is dying is not able to openly grieve or acknowledge his loss. This type of grief is
    a. Uncomplicated.
    b. Complicated.
    c. Disenfranchised.
    d. Unresolved.

136. A patient in palliative care has a 10-year-old daughter, and the patient is concerned how the child will cope with the patient's eventual death. The best advice for the patient is to
    a. Shield the child from the reality of the illness as long as possible.
    b. Ensure that the child not be involved in patient care.
    c. Send the child to live with another family member.
    d. Involve the child in patient care to the child's ability.

137. The palliative and hospice care program is developing bereavement and follow-up services for family members after patients' deaths. In order to comply with Clinical Practice Guidelines for Quality Palliative Care (guideline 3.2) of the National Consensus Project, bereavement services must be offered for a minimum period of
    a. 30 days.
    b. 90 days.
    c. 6 months.
    d. 12 months.

138. Under Element 4: Performance Improvement Projects (PIPs) of the Quality Assurance and Performance Improvement (QAPI), which entity identifies a problem to focus on?
    a. Medicare.
    b. Medicaid.
    c. Facility.
    d. State.

139. A hospice nurse routinely gives patients and family her personal telephone number and calls and visits them, even on days off, and often brings small gifts and offers to do errands. This is an example of
    a. Professional excellence.
    b. Professional boundary violation.
    c. Professional negligence.
    d. Professional inexperience.

140. The primary principle of palliative care is to
    a. Provide compassionate care.
    b. Relieve suffering.
    c. Guide the patient to acceptance of death.
    d. Respect the wishes of the person dying.

141. A nurse monitoring pain control for a palliative care patient with a history of drug abuse is concerned that the patient is exhibiting aberrant drug-taking behavior. Which of the following is of most concern?
    a. The nurse finds a rolled and partially burned fentanyl patch beside the patient's bed.
    b. The patient took one extra dose of oral pain medication.
    c. The patient changed his fentanyl patch in 2 days instead of 3.
    d. The patient complains that he needs higher doses of medication.

142. The primary difference between physician-assisted suicide and terminal sedation is
    a. There is essentially no difference.
    b. Terminal sedation is legal.
    c. Terminal sedation is intended to provide comfort and alleviate suffering.
    d. Terminal sedation does not hasten death.

143. When a patient is undergoing terminal weaning and being removed from ventilation, which medication is most indicated to relieve a sense of breathlessness?
    a. Benzodiazepine.
    b. Bronchial dilator.
    c. SSRI.
    d. Opioid.

144. According to the National Cancer Institute Scale of Severity of Diarrhea, 7 to 9 stools per day with incontinence and/or severe abdominal cramping is classified as
    a. Grade 1.
    b. Grade 2.
    c. Grade 3.
    d. Grade 4.

145. The purpose of teaching "huffing" to a patient with cystic fibrosis is to
    a. Relieve dyspnea.
    b. Improve cough effectiveness.
    c. Distract the mind.
    d. Relieve cough.

146. A patient with a fungating breast cancer tumor has tumor necrosis and a foul odor. Which treatment is most indicated to control odor?
   a. Topical metronidazole.
   b. Charcoal dressings.
   c. Topical application of yogurt.
   d. Skin cleansers.

147. When reviewing costs in relation to clinical outcomes, which of the following is based on the assumption that that two treatments are equal in effectiveness, so the least expensive option should be utilized?
   a. Cost effectiveness.
   b. Cost utility.
   c. Cost benefit.
   d. Cost minimization.

148. The three primary aspects of evidence-based practice are clinical expertise, best available research, and
   a. Patient values.
   b. Economic impact.
   c. Expected outcomes.
   d. Decision-making.

149. The primary treatment for tumor-related spinal cord compression is
   a. Corticosteroids.
   b. Decompressive therapy
   c. Fractionated external-beam radiation therapy.
   d. Analgesia.

150. In the ABCDE method of pain assessment, the E stands for
   a. Eliminate pain.
   b. Empower patients and family.
   c. Expectations.
   d. Examine patient.

Answers and Explanations

1. C: The Medicare hospice benefit is a federal program for Medicare-eligible patients with an estimated life expectancy of 6 months or less. Because Medicare is a federally funded program, eligibility requirements and benefits do not vary from state to state. The cost of all supplies and medications being used in relation to the terminal illness are covered under the Medicare hospice benefit. Hospice care may be provided in multiple settings, including home, outpatient, and inpatient settings. A patient does not need a "do not resuscitate" order to qualify for the Medicare hospice benefit. Patients who have activated the Medicare hospice benefit may opt to return to "regular" Medicare (ie, Medicare Part A) at any time.

2. B: Patients who are taking opiates long term become physically dependent on the medication and will experience symptoms of drug withdrawal if the medication is discontinued suddenly or the dose is dropped dramatically. It is important for the palliative care nurse to understand the differences between physical dependence, tolerance, and addiction to pain medications. Physical dependence occurs when the body adapts to the effects of opiate medications (taken long term) to the degree that rapid discontinuation or rapid dose decreases result in withdrawal symptoms. Tolerance to opiate medications describes the phenomenon of the body adjusting to a stable dose of medication, resulting in a need for increased amounts of the medication to achieve the same effect. Psychological dependence (or addiction) on opiate medications is characterized by a lack of control over use of the medication, compulsive use, and continued use despite harmful effects.

3. A: The essence of palliative care involves the relief of pain and suffering in the terminally ill patient. Palliative (or terminal) sedation describes the use of sedative agents (eg, benzodiazepines, barbiturates) to treat pain or suffering in the dying patient when other treatment measures are ineffective. Palliative sedation is employed to relieve intractable symptoms in the dying patient, not to expedite the dying process. Palliative sedation is somewhat controversial. Some argue that it is the ethical equivalent to euthanizing a dying patient, given that death may be hastened with the use of sedative medications. Palliative sedation is more often administered for relief of intractable physical symptoms, such as dyspnea, pain, or agitation, than for so-called "psychic" suffering. As with other decisions made in palliative care, honest discussion between providers and the patient and family members about the use of palliative sedation should occur.

4. C: The dying patient becomes progressively less mobile as his or her illness progresses. There are numerous complications associated with immobility, some of which should be prevented when possible to avoid causing discomfort in the dying patient. Complications of immobility include muscle weakness due to atrophy, constipation, joint stiffness and pain, urinary tract infection, increased clotting risk, and pressure ulcers. Pathologic fractures, myoclonus, and pruritus are commonly present in the terminally ill patient but are not increased with immobility. Pressure ulcers can be prevented or minimized with the use of turning and positioning techniques, maintenance of optimal nutritional status (when appropriate), and wound management.

5. C: Spirituality and religion may play a large part in how the terminally ill patient experiences and responds to the dying process. Assessing the role of religious or spiritual beliefs in each patient's life is an important component of a patient's assessment and should, ideally, take place as early as possible in the relationship between patient and palliative care providers. Some patients may have extensive involvement in a religious or spiritual community, while others may have deep personal beliefs, which are not necessarily associated with an official organization or community. Patients

who do not identify strongly with spiritual or religious beliefs should not be urged to do so. Spiritual and religious beliefs may influence a patient's beliefs about why they are ill, which medical interventions they are willing to pursue, rituals they would like around the time of death, and potential sources of comfort during the dying process. Although a patient's religious and spiritual beliefs may differ from the nurse's personal beliefs, the primary purpose is not to seek out differences but to discover what will be most meaningful and helpful to the patient.

6. B: Urinary incontinence is a common symptom in the palliative care patient and may significantly affect a patient's self-esteem, sexual activity, and willingness to venture out in his or her community. There are multiple causes of urinary incontinence, including urinary tract infections; limited mobility, affecting a patient's ability to get to a toilet; constipation; mental status changes; medication effects; weak pelvic floor musculature; neuropathic bladder; fistula; and poor urethral sphincter tone. Management of urinary incontinence varies greatly, depending on the cause. A patient with invasive prostate cancer causing incontinence needs treatment strategies that differ from those needed by a patient with a urinary tract infection. A thorough history, including a medication history, physical examination, and urinalysis, often reveals likely etiologies of urinary incontinence. Additionally, a bladder log, which details fluid intake, voiding, incontinence episodes, and any associated factors (eg, coughing, laughing) can be helpful in designing a management plan.

7. C: Palliative patients who have young children are often very concerned about the effect their death will have on their children. Helping a patient and his or her family feel more comfortable with assisting the children through the dying and grieving process can bring a patient a great deal of comfort. A child's understanding of illness and death and the way in which their grief is expressed often varies greatly, depending on their age and development. Many adults mistakenly believe that a young child is either unaware of the parent's illness or is unable to understand the severity of a parent's illness. Many families need and desire specific, concrete strategies for explaining the illness and death of a parent to a child. Maintaining as many of the child's usual routines as possible, answering questions directly, and encouraging the child to express any thoughts or feelings are among the helpful tips that families may need.

8. A: Pain assessment is a crucial part of palliative care nursing, and there are many different assessment tools available to the palliative care nurse for this purpose. Although not universal, pain is an extremely common symptom in the dying patient. Pain is far more than a purely physical experience for the patient, and the most effective assessment tools take into account the multiple factors that influence the individual patient's pain experience. Important factors to assess (and reassess) include specific words describing the pain; intensity (eg, 1–10 scale); location; duration; quality; associated factors; effect on sleep, appetite, mood, and energy; and the patient's attitudes or beliefs about his or her pain. Using a consistent assessment tool allows the nurse to observe trends in the patient's pain in response to therapy. Although a multifactorial assessment tool may discover adverse medication effects, withdrawal symptoms, or warning signs of psychological dependence on pain medications, most pain assessment tools are not designed for the primary assessment of these issues.

9. C: Acquired immunodeficiency syndrome (AIDS) is caused by human immunodeficiency virus (HIV), a retrovirus that primarily affects the T cells of the human immune system. T cells carry a surface protein called CD4, and the disease severity correlates with falling CD4 levels. Although the discovery and use of antiretroviral medications have markedly changed the life expectancy of most patients with HIV/AIDS, it remains a fatal illness. Because HIV affects the patient's immune system, progression of disease is primarily characterized by opportunistic infections (ie, infections that would not occur in a patient with healthy T cells). AIDS patients may also develop opportunistic

malignancies, such as Kaposi sarcoma and lymphoma, although infection is the primary cause of death in AIDS patients. Examples of opportunistic infections that occur as CD4 levels decrease include *Pneumocystis carinii* pneumonia, tuberculosis, and *Cryptococcus*. Aside from the effects of infections, AIDS patients often require end-of-life care for pain, weight loss, weakness, and mental status changes.

10. B: Although each patient's dying process is individual, the signs and symptoms of impending death are often very similar, even in patients with very different terminal illnesses. The palliative care nurse should be familiar with the common signs and symptoms of impending death so that he or she can educate the patient and caregivers about the dying process and support patients and caregivers through the patient's death. As death nears, the patient has decreasing interest in or awareness of his or her surroundings and a reduced desire or ability to move around. He or she has a marked decrease in food or fluid intake and often develops difficulty with swallowing. The dying patient usually develops noisy and irregular respirations, cool extremities, and possibly fast or irregular pulse. Urine output typically decreases or stops as the patient gets closer to dying.

11. C: Pain can be categorized in a variety of ways, and successful treatment of pain is dependent on a multidimensional and frequent assessment of the palliative care patient's pain. Treating pain well depends in part on assessing what type of pain a patient is experiencing, particularly when considering the onset and duration of action of the many different pain medications available. As the name suggests, spontaneous pain occurs spontaneously, and is not predictably associated with a particular movement or event. Incident pain is pain that occurs predictably in association with a particular event, such as walking, a dressing change, or coughing. Spontaneous pain and incident pain are different types of breakthrough pain. End-of-dose failure is pain that occurs as the time for the next dose of a scheduled pain medication approaches. In other words, the medicine is not lasting long enough. Psychic pain refers to pain that is primarily characterized by its impact on the patient's emotional state (eg, fear of dying, feeling helpless).

12. C: "Fading away" refers to the process through which patients and their loved ones go when facing a terminal illness, in which they come to terms with the change and loss that accompanies progressive illness and death. Like grief, the process of fading away may be characterized by stops and starts with multiple components of the process occurring simultaneously. "Redefining" involves making adjustments as tasks and routines in which the patient was previously able to engage in are no longer possible because of disease progression. Important nursing interventions for patients working through the redefining process include encouraging patients to express their feelings about what has changed, reminding patients of what remains possible, and assisting patients in finding new ways to engage in those activities that are meaningful to them.

13. C: Advanced practice nurses (eg, clinical nurse specialist, nurse practitioner) have completed a master's degree in nursing and maintain specialized knowledge and skills in their chosen specialty. Palliative care advanced practice nurses should be up-to-date with the latest literature and evidence-based guidelines of care. They are available both for direct patient care and education of patients, families, and other providers. They are a consultation resource in complicated or difficult cases. Administering medication for the express purpose of hastening death is not considered an appropriate palliative intervention, according to the policies of most palliative care organizations, including the American Nurses Association. This may be an evolving issue in palliative care, particularly with the passage of laws in some states that allow for the prescription of medications with the express purpose of hastening death in terminally ill patients.

14. A: Dementia is a progressive, generally irreversible disease characterized by impaired cognitive functioning, which may be caused by a variety of conditions, including AIDS, Alzheimer disease, trauma, and vascular disease. Dementia is usually a progressive disease, although specific stages of dementia are not clearly delineated. The patient in the late (ie, terminal or advanced) stage of dementia has severely impaired or complete loss of his or her ability to swallow, communicate, walk, or maintain continence. Palliative care patients with terminal dementia may experience any of the symptoms commonly seen in other terminally ill patients, including pain, infection, dyspnea, and agitation.

15. C: Superior vena cava obstruction in the palliative care patient is most commonly associated with tumors or lung cancer and results from obstruction of blood flow through the superior vena cava (SVC). Obstruction may result from either internal (eg, local cancer extension) or external (eg, bulky lymphadenopathy) compression of the SVC or may result from a clot in the SVC. Symptoms of SVC obstruction may present gradually or acutely and are often very distressing to the patient and family. The patient may complain of facial, arm, or neck swelling; shortness of breath; a feeling of fullness in the head; hoarseness; or dysphagia. Distended neck veins may be visible on examination. With rapid or complete obstruction, patients rapidly deteriorate as a result of increased intracranial pressure. Lymphedema typically results in extremity swelling, rather than facial swelling.

16. B: When terminally ill patients lack the mental capacity to make end-of-life treatment decisions, family members usually become the primary medical decision makers in the absence of a predetermined health care power of attorney. Family members may have conflicting values and opinions about end-of-life issues. Convening a family conference with palliative care providers is helpful in cases where there is disagreement among family members regarding the plan of care. Once the family members are updated about the medical status of the patient, a respectful and honest conversation should take place in which each family member's opinions and concerns about what the plan of care should be are elicited. Members of the palliative care team can encourage family members to consider what they believe the patient would have wanted if he or she were able to decide. This may be quite different from what they would choose for themselves in a similar situation.

17. A: Whether to administer artificial hydration to the dying patient should be determined within the context of the patient's symptoms and goals. Artificial (nonoral) hydration is considered a medical intervention in the United States, and its use can, therefore, be refused if the patient or care team feels its burdens outweigh the benefits. Family members and care providers may find it emotionally difficult not to provide artificial hydration to the dying patient. Dehydration that occurs as patients reduce their oral fluid intake may lead to improvement in some end-of-life symptoms, such as edema, vomiting, and respiratory congestion. Dehydration is not typically associated with pain in most patients. In some patients, dehydration may exacerbate distressing end-of-life symptoms, such as delirium from electrolyte abnormalities, or impaired consciousness from poor clearance of sedating medications (eg, opiates). Patients with decision-making capacity can make informed decisions to accept or refuse artificial hydration.

18. D: The sensation of dry mouth (xerostomia) is a common complaint in the palliative care patient and can lead to discomfort as well as difficulty with chewing, swallowing, speaking, and taste. Xerostomia can result in mouth sores, halitosis, and dental decay. Treatment can prevent complications of xerostomia and provides increased patient comfort. Xerostomia may occur for a variety of reasons, including decreased saliva secretion, damage to the buccal mucosa, dehydration, and psychological factors. Many medications used in palliative care (eg, anticholinergic medications), oxygen therapy, and mouth breathing also contribute to dry mouth. There are

- 103 -

multiple treatment options for xerostomia once underlying conditions have been treated (if possible). Nonpharmacologic therapies include basic mouth care (eg, lip/mouth swabs, toothbrushing), peppermint water, vitamin C, gum or mints, and acupuncture. Pharmacologic therapies include artificial saliva solutions, pilocarpine, bethanechol, and yohimbine. Although topical anesthetic may be helpful for treating painful mouth sores, it is not a primary treatment for xerostomia.

19. D: Opioid medications are commonly used by terminally ill patients and are highly effective for treatment of pain. Long-term opioid use is often accompanied by unpleasant side effects. The goal should be to find a treatment regimen that treats the patient's pain adequately while minimizing uncomfortable or distressing side effects. Sedation is a common side effect of opiate medications. The somnolence associated with opiate administration often improves or resolves within 1 to 2 days of starting the medication. If sedation continues, it is important to review other potential causes, including other central nervous system depressant medications (eg, benzodiazepines). If the patient is without pain, reducing the opiate dose may be effective. If the patient is unable to tolerate a reduced opiate dose, psychostimulant medications (eg, methylphenidate) can be effective.

20. D: Poverty presents additional challenges to providing optimal palliative care to the terminally ill patient. Often, patients living in poverty have unstable (or nonexistent) housing, making it difficult to provide "home" care consistently. Lack of telephone access and dependable transportation options lead to difficulty with arranging or getting to scheduled or urgent medical visits. Patients may be dealing with the challenges of meeting their most basic needs, such as food and shelter. Patients living in poverty may not have a stable support system, leading to lack of a friend or family member who can function as a caregiver as illness progresses. If the patient is dealing with addiction or psychiatric illness in addition to poverty, the challenges are significantly compounded. Contrary to popular stereotypes, patients living in poverty do not necessarily have less effective coping skills. As with all patients, there is a wide range of psychological reactions to end-of-life issues, and many patients who are homeless or struggling to meet their basic needs on a day-to-day basis are resilient, flexible, and pragmatic when faced with the challenge of terminal illness.

21. B: Pain is a common symptom in terminally ill patients, but there are different types of pain, and different therapies are more effective with certain types of pain than with others. Physiologic or sensory pain is generally classified into three categories. Neuropathic pain is fairly localized (but radiating) pain that arises from nerve infiltration or injury (eg, tumor infiltration, postherpetic neuralgia) and is often described as shooting, burning, tingling, or shock-like. Somatic pain is well-localized pain that arises from stimulation of skin, bone, or muscle (eg, bony metastases, cellulitis) and is often described as achy, throbbing, or dull. Visceral pain is poorly localized pain that arises from stimulation of abdominal or thoracic viscera (eg, ischemic bowel, hepatic capsule distention) and is often described as cramping, squeezing, or pressure.

22. A: Hope is an important component of life, even as people face terminal illness and death, and is an adaptive and healthy response to life's challenges. Assisting patients in maintaining hope in the face of terminal illness and impending death is an important tool of the palliative care provider. "False hope" (or "unrealistic hopefulness" or denial) is somewhat controversial among palliative care providers and family members of terminally ill patients. Some providers feel that any attachment to unrealistic hopes is unhealthy and indicative of impaired coping. As with other assessments in palliative care nursing, one can assess a patient's "unrealistic hopes" to establish whether the patient's beliefs and hopes are causing any actual harm. Gentle intervention may be

warranted if the patient's beliefs and hopes are leading to risky behaviors, refusal to seek crucial medical care, or social isolation. In the absence of demonstrated harm to the patient, it should be acknowledged that denial is a legitimate coping mechanism, and patients should not be pushed to accept their impending death until they feel ready to do so.

23. C: Delirium is a complex and common clinical phenomenon in the palliative care patient and is characterized by "acute and fluctuating disturbances in attention, level of consciousness, and basic cognitive functions," according to the *Diagnostic and Statistical Manual of Mental Disorders* (Fourth Edition). Patients may be disoriented, agitated, and hallucinating. Patients with delirium may have increased psychomotor activity (eg, sleep disturbance, agitation, loud speech, combative), decreased psychomotor activity (eg, lethargy, apathy), or a combination of the two. Although there are overlapping features of delirium and dementia (eg, mood lability, memory disturbances), the time course and fluctuating nature of delirium differentiates it from dementia. Dementia is a slow-onset progressive disease, occurring over months and years, as opposed to hours and days. Palliative care patients are at increased risk for delirium because of their serious medical illness and multiple medications.

24. A: The Medicare hospice benefit is a federal program for Medicare-eligible patients with an estimated life expectancy of 6 months or less. The cost of all supplies and medications being used in relation to the terminal illness is covered. The Medicare hospice benefit covers inpatient respite care for up to 5 consecutive days to provide short-term relief to a hospice patient's primary caregiver. Additionally, the Medicare hospice benefit covers routine home care, inpatient care for medical conditions or complications related to the terminal illness, and continuous home care for medical complications that would otherwise require inpatient hospitalization.

25. B: Noninvasive positive pressure ventilation (eg, BiPAP) may be utilized in the palliative care setting for relief of dyspnea in some patients or for patients who do not wish to be intubated for respiratory failure but would like more aggressive intervention than supplemental oxygen. As with all interventions in palliative care, the benefits of a particular therapy for meeting the patient's end-of-life goals must be weighed against the burdens of therapy. In patients with ALS whose dyspnea and respiratory failure is due to a primary weakness in the respiratory muscles, BiPAP has been shown to improve quality of life and prolong survival. Of course, many patients with ALS choose not to use BiPAP or choose to discontinue BiPAP if its use is no longer meeting their goals for end-of-life care. The use of BiPAP is not a contraindication for the administration of medications commonly used to relieve dyspnea in the dying patient.

26. C: Lymphedema is a distressing and difficult-to-treat edema secondary to impaired drainage of lymphatic fluid. Lymphedema typically occurs in an extremity and is characterized by swelling, skin tightness, variable discomfort, decreased range of motion, and skin changes, such as weeping or thickening. Breast cancer patients who have undergone surgery with dissection of the axillary lymph nodes or radiation therapy account for the most common source of upper extremity lymphedema, although lymphedema may also be associated with other cancers, infection, trauma, or thrombosis. Treatment is long term and may include manual lymphatic drainage, compression devices, skin care, and treatment of underlying conditions, when possible.

27. A: Fentanyl is a highly potent opioid medication, which can be administered in multiple forms, including intravenously, subcutaneously, and transdermally. Transdermal fentanyl is beneficial in palliative care patients who can no longer take oral medications safely or are experiencing intractable vomiting. The analgesic effects of transdermal fentanyl last about 72 hours, but analgesic effect and steady-state serum levels are delayed until at least 12 hours after the patch is applied. Absorption may be altered by patient factors, such as body habitus or fever. External heat

applied over a fentanyl patch may increase the rate of medication absorption. Given the slow onset and offset of transdermally absorbed fentanyl, this route is not appropriate or effective for the treatment of breakthrough pain.

28. A: One of the essential tenets of palliative care is respect for the patient's right to make independent, well-informed choices about his or her life and death. However, one of the most effective tools that a patient has for ensuring that his or her wishes are respected as death approaches, the health care power of attorney or medical advance directive, is underused. There are misconceptions both among health care providers and patients and families that impede the use of these legal avenues for maintaining control over medical decision making. Ideally, discussions with patients about advance directives should occur either before serious illness develops or before the terminal phase of an existing illness. Some providers mistakenly believe that bringing up this topic with patients will scare them, but research demonstrates that most patients prefer to be asked about these issues early on. Some patients mistakenly believe that an advance directive makes it less likely that they will receive advanced medical treatment. Patients need to be assured that they will retain full medical decision-making power unless and until they are no longer able to do so.

29. B: Malodorous malignant wounds create a great deal of distress for patients and families and may result in a patient feeling isolated or ashamed. Suggesting and providing therapeutic options for minimizing wound odor is an important service that the palliative care nurse can provide to assist the patient in maintaining his or her dignity as death approaches. The most common cause of wound odor is colonization with anaerobic bacteria. Treatment and prevention strategies include regular wound cleaning, debridement of necrotic tissue, topical metronidazole application, and charcoal dressings or odor-absorbing charcoal in the patient's room. Topical steroids are not indicated for treatment of wound odor. Calcium alginate dressings are used to control bleeding in wounds. Systemic metronidazole use is not indicated for treatment of local wound colonization.

30. C: Patients and family members can have a wide range of adaptive and healthy coping styles, depending on their personality, past experience, and cultural factors. Caregivers of a terminally ill patient experience a great deal of stress and fatigue as they deal with the physical challenges of a progressively sicker loved one and the emotional strain of the impending death of a family member. It is important for the palliative care nurse to assess and assist the patient's caregivers in the often monumental tasks that accompany caring for a dying loved one. Signs that may indicate unhealthy or impaired coping of a patient's caregivers include expressing almost exclusively "negative" feelings (eg, anger), withholding information from other family members, refusing to accept assistance, focusing exclusively on their own needs, or refusing to acknowledge or accommodate differences in opinion among caregivers. The palliative care nurse who has taken the time to become familiar with the strengths and weaknesses of the patient's loved ones can often recognize impaired coping and intervene early with appropriate support and resources.

31. C: Pain is a common symptom in terminally ill patients, and many misconceptions and barriers exist that interfere with both adequate assessment and treatment of a patient's pain. Inadequate or overly narrow pain assessment tools, provider prejudices, mistrust between patient and provider, concerns about addiction to pain medication, and cultural variations in communicating pain are just some of the common barriers to adequate pain treatment. Patients may underreport pain for a variety of reasons, such as attempting to avoid side effects of pain medication, concern about hastening death, or family expectations about stoicism in the face of pain. It is important for providers to review the difference between psychological dependence and physical dependence on

- 106 -

pain medications if a patient or family member voices concern about drug addiction in the context of analgesic therapy.

32. B: It is important for the palliative care nurse to be familiar with organizational positions and guidelines surrounding common end-of-life issues. The American Nurses Association (ANA) position on artificial hydration and nutrition in the terminally ill patient states that decisions to forgo artificial hydration or nutrition in association with end-of-life care should be made by the patient and the health care team. Artificial (nonoral) hydration is considered a medical intervention in the United States, and its use can, therefore, be refused if the patient or care team feels its burdens outweigh the benefits. Dehydration is not typically associated with pain or discomfort in the dying patient. The position of the ANA on active euthanasia and assisted suicide states that it is in conflict with the ethical and professional traditions and goals of a nurse to participate in either active euthanasia or assisted suicide. This may evolve as states pass legislation that allows terminally ill patients to pursue medications administered with the express purpose of hastening death.

33. A: Caring for patients with terminal illness and their families through the dying process inevitably elicits strong emotional responses in the palliative care nurse. Palliative care nurses become intimately involved with patients and their families and deal with the loss of patient after patient as his or her professional experience grows. Just as patients and families experience nonlinear progression through the grieving and adaptation process, so do palliative care nurses. One model of hospice nurse adjustment (formulated by Bernice Harper) describes five progressive stages: intellectualization, emotional survival, depression, emotional arrival, and deep compassion. Hospice nurses must have both institutional and individual support systems and strategies in place to engage effectively in self-care and to provide the best care for their patients.

34. A: Constipation is an unpleasant and common symptom in the palliative care patient, and the etiology is often multifactorial. It is important for the palliative care nurse to anticipate and regularly screen for constipation in the terminally ill patient. Constipation can cause abdominal or rectal pain, leakage of liquid stool, urinary retention, and agitation. Common contributing factors to constipation in the hospice patient include medications (especially opiates), reduced mobility, reduced fluid intake, mechanical obstruction because of tumor or spinal cord compression, and metabolic derangements (eg, hypercalcemia or hypokalemia). *Clostridium difficile* infection typically causes diarrhea rather than constipation.

35. D: Neuropathic pain is not particularly well understood and is difficult to treat. Neuropathic pain does not respond to nonsteroidal anti-inflammatory drugs or opiate medications as reliably as other types of pain. The drug treatment of choice for neuropathic pain is antidepressant medication, generally tricyclics (eg, amitriptyline) or selective serotonin reuptake inhibitors (eg, paroxetine). Onset of analgesic effects with tricyclic antidepressants is generally within 3 to 4 days of beginning the medication, as opposed to the several weeks it typically takes for depressive symptom relief. Adverse effects frequently occur with use of tricyclic antidepressants. Tricyclic antidepressants are not indicated or effective for non-neuropathic pain (aside from so-called "psychic pain") in the palliative care patient.

36. C: Interdisciplinary palliative care teams ensure that providers from multiple specialties (eg, physician, social worker, nurse, chaplain) can collaborate with the patient and family to craft a care plan that meets the needs and goals of the patient. Care is directed primarily by the patient. Ideally, the team provides information and elicits patient values, preferences, and goals as they pertain to end-of-life care. Once this is completed, specific challenges can be identified and possible solutions

planned. Interventions are then provided for the patient and family in accordance with the formulated plan. Reassessments and changes in the care plan are made as illness progresses or preferences or goals change.

37. D: Bowel obstruction in the hospice patient is most commonly seen in the patient with ovarian or bowel cancer due to primary tumor or peritoneal metastasis. Bowel obstruction typically presents with abdominal pain and vomiting. Treatment may consist primarily of palliative symptom management with antiemetics and pain medications. Antisecretory medications or promotility agents may be helpful for symptom management in some patients. If the patient wishes to pursue more aggressive treatment, it may be appropriate to provide intravenous hydration, nasogastric tube placement, gastrostomy placement, or surgical intervention.

38. C: Many patients with terminal illness explore and pursue complementary and alternative therapies to treat either their primary disease or side effects associated with treatment. Nausea and vomiting are very disruptive and unpleasant for most patients, and may be difficult to manage, particularly when medications being used to treat other symptoms (eg, pain) contribute to nausea and vomiting. Acupuncture is one of the alternative medicine therapies, in addition to massage, progressive muscle relaxation, and meditation, that has been shown to be effective in managing nausea and vomiting in patients with chronic illnesses. Although some complementary and alternative therapies are not proven to help with symptoms, the only good reason to discourage a palliative care patient from exploring other therapeutic modalities is if the therapy is either unsafe or interacts negatively with other treatment the patient is receiving.

39. D: Dyspnea (shortness of breath) is a common and distressing symptom in terminally ill patients, particularly patients with chronic obstructive pulmonary disease, heart failure, respiratory muscle weakness, or pulmonary pathology from cancer. General supportive measures for treatment of dyspnea include upright positioning, placement near an open window or fan, relaxation techniques, and supplemental oxygen administration. The drug treatment of choice for treating persistent dyspnea is opiates. Depending on the etiology and progression of dyspnea, benzodiazepines, glycopyrrolate, steroids, diuretics, or bronchodilators may also be helpful.

40. A: Pain is a multifactorial sensation, encompassing physiologic and sensory components in addition to psychological, spiritual, and social components. Ideally, the palliative care nurse makes use of a valid and consistent multidimensional pain assessment tool. The factors described by this patient encompass physiologic and sensory components of her pain, such as quality, location, duration, intensity, and alleviating or aggravating factors. A description encompassing psychological or affective aspects of pain may include a report of the patient's emotional experience with regard to the pain, particular ways in which the patient expresses pain, and the impact of the pain on the patient's mood. Sociocultural aspects of pain that may be assessed include impact of the pain on the patient's role in his or her family, job, and cultural community.

41. B: It is critically important for palliative care nurses to be aware of the relative potencies of different opiate medications and to understand how to calculate equianalgesic doses of opioids when changing from one opiate medication to another. There are readily available conversion charts for the palliative care nurse to consult when calculating the appropriate dosage of a new opioid. Administration route also needs to be taken into account when calculating drug dosages. The palliative care nurse may be converting the same medication from one route to another (eg, parenteral to oral), may be changing the drug without changing the route of administration (eg, parenteral hydromorphone replacing parenteral morphine), or may be changing both the medication and the route (eg, parenteral morphine to oral hydrocodone). Hydromorphone is more

potent than morphine. A 1.5 mg dose of parenteral hydromorphone is equianalgesic to a 10 mg dose of parenteral morphine.

42. B: The Medicare hospice benefit provides for four different levels of hospice care, depending on the needs of the terminally ill patient. Routine home care (most common) is provided wherever the patient lives (eg, private home, long-term care facility). Respite care consists of up to 5 consecutive days of inpatient hospice care to provide relief to a family caregiver. General inpatient hospice care is provided for the patient whose home environment is no longer a safe environment or the patient who is having intractable symptoms that are unmanageable in the home setting. Finally, continuous home care is available for patients who would like to remain in their homes but are having symptoms that would otherwise require inpatient hospice care. In this case, inpatient hospice care is essentially brought to the patient in their home setting.

43. D: An important component of palliative nursing, particularly if a patient will remain in a home setting, is education of caregivers. Depending on the clinical situation, caregivers may need to learn when and how to administer medications, wound care, patient movement and positioning techniques, and symptoms that commonly develop as the patient nears death. Although the coping skills and cognitive abilities of patient caregivers vary, a very effective technique for solidifying caregiver learning and allowing the nurse to assess the learning is to have the caregiver demonstrate what they have been taught. With turning and positioning maneuvers taught for pressure ulcer prevention, it is most helpful for the caregiver to demonstrate the learned maneuvers with the actual patient.

44. B: There are many different forms of complementary and alternative medicine that palliative care patients may choose to explore at different stages of their illness. These may include Chinese herbs, homeopathy, hypnosis, specialized diets, biofeedback, massage, guided imagery, naturopathy, vitamin supplements, meditation, art and music therapy, chiropractic manipulation, acupuncture, and energy therapies. Therapeutic touch refers to the use of touch, while healing and positive energy is directed to the patient. Yoga involves body poses and breathing techniques to facilitate relaxation and healing. Reflexology involves stimulation of areas of the hands, feet, and ears, which are believed to correspond to different body parts and organ systems. It is helpful for the palliative care nurses to familiarize themselves with complementary therapies that patients may be interested in using.

45. D: Although tricyclic antidepressants are one of the few therapies that may be effective for treatment of neuropathic pain, they have a high incidence of adverse effects. Anticholinergic effects are common, and include dry mouth, urinary retention, tachycardia, delirium, and constipation. Other adverse effects associated with tricyclic antidepressant use include cardiac arrhythmias, sedation, weight gain, sweating, and sexual dysfunction. Patients may be unwilling to continue taking these medications if adverse effects are more distressing than the symptoms for which they are being used to treat.

46. C: Heart failure results in fluid overload, leading to pulmonary edema, hepatic congestion, and peripheral edema. Dyspnea is a common symptom, primarily from pulmonary edema. Patients with severe heart failure also commonly have pain (ie, chest, extremity or abdominal pain from ischemia and congestion), dysrhythmias, fatigue, sexual dysfunction, anorexia, and depression. Treatment and palliation for symptoms of heart failure may include oxygen, antiarrhythmics, antidepressants, and analgesic medication. Diuretics are commonly administered to manage symptoms that are caused by fluid overload, including pulmonary edema. Dyspnea often improves when patients with heart failure are treated with diuretics, because pulmonary fluid overload is decreased.

47. D: Feelings of sadness and anxiety are normal and appropriate reactions in response to a grave prognosis. Normal adjustment reactions and grief can be difficult to differentiate from depression and anxiety disorders. In general, normal grieving and depression are differentiated by the severity and duration of symptoms, as well as by the degree to which symptoms are interfering with other aspects of the patient's life or relationships. Features that are expected with normal grief include sadness, anger, worry, fear, and potentially some degree of temporary social withdrawal. Features that would be more concerning for a psychiatric diagnosis, such as depression or anxiety, include hopelessness, suicidal ideation, and poor self-image. The palliative care nurse should continue to support and assess a patient through the grieving process so that the patient can be further evaluated or treated with counseling or psychiatric medication as needed.

48. B: Myoclonic jerks are sudden, brief, and uncontrollable movements. They most commonly occur in an extremity. Myoclonus can be very distressing to the palliative care patient and family members and may be uncomfortable or exhausting. Myoclonus is most commonly caused by opiate medications in the palliative care patient. Generally, myoclonus is considered a sign of opiate toxicity and is an indication for changing to a different opiate medication. Providers may also use opiate antagonists, such as naloxone, for acute treatment of myoclonus. Changing to a different opiate often results in resolution of myoclonus. Benzodiazepines and antispasmodics are used for treatment of myoclonus in some patients.

49. D: Noisy breathing is very common in the dying patient, and generally indicates that death is imminent (within hours). Although most patients who have the "death rattle" have a diminished level of consciousness and are not distressed by the respiratory congestion, it can be quite distressing to loved ones when a patient's respirations are loud and appear labored. The "death rattle" is due to pooling of oral and respiratory secretions in the pharynx and upper airways as the airway protective reflexes diminish. If the patient or family desires treatment, the first-line treatment is anticholinergic medications, such as scopolamine, atropine, and glycopyrrolate. This often diminishes the volume of secretions. Repositioning the patient may also improve symptoms. Suctioning can be uncomfortable and lead to patient agitation and is, therefore, not generally recommended unless the patient is essentially comatose.

50. B: Hypercalcemia is an urgent and serious complication of late-stage malignancy (unrelated to bone metastases) with a significant mortality rate if untreated. Hypercalcemia most commonly occurs in the setting of breast cancer and multiple myeloma but may occur with other malignancies as well. Symptoms of hypercalcemia can be somewhat nonspecific and include gastrointestinal symptoms (eg, nausea, vomiting, constipation, anorexia), neurologic symptoms (eg, weakness, mental status changes, fatigue), and cardiac symptoms (eg, bradycardia, electrocardiogram changes). Treatment, if in keeping with the goals of the palliative care patient, includes intravenous hydration for correction of dehydration, calcitonin (inhibits bone resorption and facilitates calcium excretion), and bisphosphonates. Bisphosphonates are very effective at inhibiting bone resorption and reducing serum calcium levels, but their calcium-lowering effects are delayed until about 48 hours after administration.

51. D: Patients with some types of cancer complain of a very bad taste in the mouth, but some strategies may help increase input:
Avoid highly spiced foods.
Avoid hot foods and avoid being in the kitchen when food is prepared if possible.
Rinse the mouth with a salt and soda mixture before eating.
Use a straw to drink liquids to minimize contact with taste buds.

Drink very cold liquids and eat cold or room temperature food instead of hot.

52. B: Fecal impaction occurs when the hard stool moves into the rectum and becomes a large, dense, immovable mass that cannot be evacuated even with straining, usually as a result of chronic constipation. In addition to abdominal cramps and distention, the person may feel intense rectal pressure and pain accompanied by a sense of urgency to defecate. Nausea and vomiting may also occur. Hemorrhoids will often become engorged. Fecal incontinence, with liquid stool leaking around the impaction, is common. An impaction may cause pressure on the bladder neck, obstructing urinary flow, resulting in overflow incontinence.

53. A: Visceral pain frequently requires opioids to control it, although in early stages of disease when pain is less severe, patients may respond to NSAIDs. Neuropathic pain often responds poorly to opioids and is better treated with antidepressants, anticonvulsants, and/or benzodiazepines. Somatic pain may be treated with various drugs, including steroids, NSAIDs, muscle relaxants, and bisphosphonates. Psychological pain is usually treated with psychiatric treatment that may or may not include the use of psychotropic drugs.

54. C: "Caregiving is very difficult and exhausting" reflects back what the daughter is saying about the demands for care without being judgmental and/or making her feel guilty. In fact, caregivers often feel some relief mixed with grief when a family member has died because the constant anxiety of anticipating death and providing care is extremely stressful, and reassuring the daughter that her feelings are normal can help to alleviate any guilt she might feel.

55. A: When initiating a delicate discussion about ending treatment, the best approach is to be direct but avoid trying to influence the decision directly: "Do you want to continue dialysis?" The nurse should avoid statements that suggest there is "nothing more we can do" or "we have exhausted all remedies" but should stress the things that can be done, such as providing adequate medication for pain relief and positioning the patient for comfort. Pointing out that a treatment is "prolonging" suffering may make family members feel guilty and distressed.

56. B: Federal law requires that family decision makers be asked about organ donations when patients die in the hospital if there is no advance directive outlining the patient's wishes. In many cases, patients are provided information about organ donation on admission to the hospital. Staff is not legally required to ask about donations if a patient dies at home because organs are often not viable and the deceased may be taken directly to a funeral home. The spouse is usually the family decision maker; if there is no spouse but multiple children, conflicts can arise.

57. D: Three tests are used to assess for the presence of xerostomia:
Cracker test: The patient is given a dry cracker to eat. If the patient is unable to chew and swallow the cracker without drinking liquid, then the test is positive.
Tongue blade test: A tongue blade is placed flat on a patient's tongue. Because xerostomia results in pasty thickened saliva, if the tongue blade sticks to the tongue, the test is positive.
Measurement of saliva (stimulated or unstimulated): Mouth is swabbed or patient spits repeatedly into a container for a set amount of time.

58. C: The best approach is to prepare the daughter with, "Let's talk about what to expect and what to do," because people are often fearful about death, especially if they are unsure what to expect. Death is not always predictable, so assuring the daughter that the hospice nurse will be with her or that she can transfer her father to the hospital is not truthful. The nurse should avoid platitudes,

such as "I'm sure you'll be fine," because that doesn't address the daughter's concerns and is not helpful.

59. B: Antihypertensives and other drugs that do not directly contribute to patient comfort are usually discontinued in the final days. These include diuretics, antibiotics, hormones, antidysrhythmics, hypoglycemic agents, and laxatives. Medications that are usually continued as long as possible include sedatives and analgesics. When indicated to control symptoms, other medications that are continued include antipyretics, antiemetics, anticholinergics, and anticonvulsants. Oral medications can be continued as long as a patient can swallow, often in liquid form rather than pills or capsules. Other medications may be administered parenterally.

60. D: Because the patient remains conscious and adverse effects of abrupt discontinuation of corticosteroids can be severe, the medication should be discontinued after tapering. Corticosteroids are commonly given to patients with brain tumors to reduce cerebral edema and intracranial pressure in order to control pain and seizures; therefore, as the corticosteroid dose is tapered, the dosage of anticonvulsant should be increased as the risk of seizures will increase. Analgesia may also need to be increased because the patient may experience more headaches.

61. B: All of these are indications that the patient is nearing death, but lack of radial pulse indicates that the death is likely to occur within a few hours because the strength of cardiac compressions has lessened considerably. As patients with cardiorespiratory disease near death, the pulse rate often doubles and dysrhythmias occur, as well as decreased strength of compressions. Cyanosis may be evident in nail beds, knees, and tip of nose. Mottling of the extremities usually begins to occur within a few days of death.

62. C: As patients near death, they are unable to cough to clear secretions that begin to pool in the oropharynx and bronchi, resulting in rales, usually referred to as "death rattles." Because the sound is often distressing to family members, an anticholinergic, such as glycopyrrolate or atropine, may be given subcutaneously to relieve respiratory distress. A hyoscine hydrobromide transdermal patch is also available, but action is slower, 12 hours compared with 1 minute for injections. Elevating the head of the bed or turning the patient to the side may also relieve rattling.

63. A: Palliative care should be provided to patients with life-threatening diseases throughout the disease process and continuum of care because patients need support and often adequate pain management even in earlier stages of disease. Palliative care can provide emotional and spiritual support to help patients during curative treatments and to prepare the patient and family members for the inevitable decline in health and help them to make decisions and plan for the type of supportive care that best fits their wishes.

64. D: Under the Medicare benefit, caregivers are allowed respite care periodically. Respite care is in-patient care for a period of not more than 5 days, usually in a long-term care facility or hospice facility. In this case, the husband can be provided care to allow his caregiver time to rest and decide on other options, such as hiring an assistant if finances allow. Providing daily nursing visits does little to relieve the time-consuming work of caregiving.

65. C: The CMS regulations regarding the Medicare Hospice Benefit include the requirement that an interdisciplinary team providing hospice care must include at least a physician, nurse, counselor, and social worker, but this does not preclude members from additional medical specialties, such as a nutritionist or occupational therapist. The interdisciplinary team should meet regularly to discuss

patient needs and should have easy access to data, such as laboratory studies, to help plan patient care. The use of good communication strategies among team members is critical.

66. D: Byock and Merriman's end-of-life construct includes 6 dimensions, all of which apply to both patient and caregiver:
Well-being: Subjective feelings about condition and emotions, including anxiety, fear, readiness, and acceptance.
Physical: Comfort level and physical distress.
Function: Ability to carry out activities of daily living (ADL).
Interpersonal: Degree and quality of relationships and changes resulting from caregiving.
Transcendent: Perception of meaning of life, as well as spiritual and/or religious values.
A change in one dimension will have an effect on the other dimensions, for example, an increase in pain may result in decreased ability to function, increased fear and anxiety, stress on relationships, and spiritual conflict.

67. A: One of the tasks associated with accepting the finality of life is emotional withdrawal (decathexis). Other tasks include accepting the need for dependency and acknowledging and expressing feelings of personal loss and impending death. Another landmark is recognition of a "new" self, which includes accepting a new personal definition of self and recognizing that the new self has value. Finding a sense of personal meaning for life includes completing a life review and sharing stories and information with others. Experiencing personal love of self includes being able to forgive and acknowledge oneself.

68. B: While listening to the patient's life review strengthens the personal relationship between the patient and the caregiver, it does not necessarily imply acceptance of the finality of life. As caregivers begin to accept that death is inevitable and final, they may begin to experience anticipatory grief not only for the loss of the patient but also other losses that may ensue, such as loss of financial support and social relationships. Caregivers may be able to articulate personal loss and still be able to tell the patient that it is all right to let go and die.

69. B: Stage II, emotional survival. Stages of adaptation:
I, Intellectualism (0-3 months): Focus on intellectualism and may feel anxiety while learning policies and procedures and experience superficial acceptance.
II, Emotional survival (3-6 months): May overidentify with patient's situation and experience increasing discomfort, guilt, and sadness but have increasing emotional involvement.
III, Depression (6-9 months): Less intellectualism but more grief, discomfort, and depression, overidentifying with the patient personally.
IV, Emotional arrival (9-12 months): Interactions with patient/family healthy and productive and effectively coping with loss.
V, Deep compassion (1-2 years): Acceptance of death/loss and able to express compassion and provide care with respect and dignity.

70. C: "I'm so sorry you had to experience discomfort" acknowledges the patient's concern and expresses empathy and support without making excuses or placing blame on the patient or the technician. Patients who are coming to terms with a life-threatening illness often exhibit emotional lability and may experience profound, undifferentiated anger, lashing out at others. They may take this anger out on family members and care providers, overreacting and sometimes fixating on what they consider ill treatment.

71. B: A normal response to grief is to cry, but crying uncontrollably or not at all is often an indication of depression. With normal grief, people experience loss recurrently and may be preoccupied with loss and experience emotional lability, openly expressing anger. They have difficulty sleeping and have vivid, distressing dreams. They may have a loss of energy and mild, weight loss. Depression tends to persist with people in a constant state of unhappiness. Insomnia or hypersomnia without dreaming is common as are extreme lack of energy and pronounced weight loss. People may isolate themselves and show little emotion.

72. B: "It must be very difficult to believe what is happening to your husband" provides support to the caregiver without directly challenging the person's need to utilize denial to deal with the loss. Denial is very common, both for patients and caregivers. Some patients, for example, resist having laboratory or radiographic studies done because they do not want to know the results. Caregivers may express frustration with patients who aren't "trying" hard enough or may try to force patients to eat or take treatments.

73. D: The best response is, "Tell me why you feel you want to die now," because this encourages the patient to express his feelings without being judgmental or citing legal issues. Many patients who want to die feel that way because of uncontrolled pain or other symptoms or unresolved issues, such as depression. If the nurse can find out what is motivating the patient to consider suicide, then the nurse can often help to find a better solution.

74. A: Children in the preoperational stage (ages 2 to 7) often develop magical thinking, believing that something they have said or done can cause harm or illness to someone, especially if the children have said "I hate you" or "I wish you were dead," because they believe that their words have power of creation. Young children may fear being abandoned. Adolescents may express anger and become withdrawn and uncooperative. They may have difficulty concentrating, so grades may suffer.

75. B: When making a death pronouncement, the nurse should always first acknowledge the family and introduce himself/herself. The nurse should always check the patient for heart sounds and breath sounds even though the patient may appear deceased. Once the nurse is assured the patient is, in fact, deceased, then the nurse should confirm the death with family members and express condolences. The nurse should ask the next of kin (usually spouse or child) about autopsy and organ donation (if appropriate) and which funeral home to contact. The nurse should notify the physician of the patient's death.

76. D: Patients with advanced disease often become exhausted from treatments, adverse effects, and emotional ups and downs, leading to depression. Patients who are severely depressed should always be assessed for suicidal ideation by directly asking them if they have considered hurting themselves and if they have a plan. While acceptance of inevitable death is a normal progression, wanting to die because of depression is different from acceptance. Depressed patients may need referral for counseling and may benefit from antidepressants.

77. C: A strong religious faith often provides comfort to surviving family members and helps them cope with grief. Risk factors for complicated bereavement include a history of substance abuse or mental illness, recent loss of another family member or close friend or associate, concurrent crisis, severe anxiety or anger, concurrent illnesses, difficult death, absence of religious/spiritual belief, lack of adequate support system, and anticipated problems, such as change in economic status. Age may also be a factor, especially with surviving children.

78. B: "What positive memory do you have of raising your children" encourages the woman to think differently about her experience as a mother and can lead to a discussion of what she felt she had done right and wrong. Later in the discussion, the nurse might ask the patient to imagine what she might have done differently, although this may be a painful question for some. Platitudes, such as "I'm sure you did the best you could," are not helpful. Patient's concerns should never be dismissed with statements like, "That's not important now."

79. D: Nurses should not stereotype people based on appearance. Concerns about diversion should center on the patient. Indications include a sudden change in response to pain medications that had been controlling pain well and a difference in the appearance of pain medications (size, shape, color). Patients may also have a pattern of more analgesia use with some caregivers than others, suggesting that records may be falsified. Caregivers who are diverting drugs often begin to isolate patients, refusing home care and missing doctor's appointments.

80. A: Both Islam and Orthodox Judaism consider embalming a desecration of the body. Hindus and Buddhists are usually cremated and have no need for embalming. There is, in fact, no valid health and safety reason for embalming, and it is rarely practiced outside of the United States and Canada. If burial is to be delayed, then the body must be kept refrigerated if it is not embalmed. No state requires embalming (although 3 states require embalming if bodies are transported across state lines), and funeral directors must advise clients of this.

81. B: Because the patient is taking frequent pain pills and is forgetful, probably the best solution is to switch to a fentanyl patch because it will maintain a stable level of pain control and only needs to be changed every 3 days. However, it may take 2 to 3 days after initial application of the patch to reach the maximum level of pain control, so the patient may need to supplement with oral tablets. After that, the tablets may be used for breakthrough pain.

82. D: Because the patient's medication dosage has been increased, one can assume a comprehensive pain assessment was done initially, so at this time the only necessary assessment is of the intensity of pain with the 0 to 10 scale, with 0 indicating no pain and 10 the worst possible pain, in order to evaluate the patient's response to the dosage change. Alternate intensity scales may be used for young children or nonresponsive or confused older children or adults.

83. A: The 5 key elements of pain assessment include the following:
Words: Used to describe pain, such as burning, stabbing, deep, shooting, and sharp. Some may complain of pressure, squeezing, and discomfort rather than pain.
Intensity: Use of 0-10 scale or other appropriate scale to quantify the degree of pain.
Location: Where patient indicates pain.
Duration: Constant or comes and goes, breakthrough pain.
Aggravating/Alleviating factors: Those things that increase the intensity of pain and those that relieve the pain.

84. A: Visceral pain may occur with ascites, bowel obstruction, and hepatic cancer, and is often poorly localized and described as cramping, distention ("bloated"), deep, squeezing, and stretching. Neuropathic pain may occur with postherpetic neuralgia and diabetic neuropathy, and is described as burning, shooting, and numb or pins and needles. Somatic pain may occur from bone metastases, fractures, and arthritis, and tends to be localized and described as dull, aching, throbbing, and sore. Psychological pain related to psychological disorders is often described as affecting the entire body.

85. B: Because the patient is able to keep a record of pain medications, the patient is probably not confused or giving the medication to someone else. However, patients are often reluctant to admit the degree of pain and minimize their discomfort when asked about their pain, so it is important to determine how much pain medication the patient is actually taking and to observe the patient's behavior for indications of pain. Some patients may believe that having pain indicates their condition is poor and persist in saying they have little pain despite obvious evidence otherwise.

86. A: When the hospice movement first began, there were fewer choices for analgesia, and the use of morphine or "morphine cocktails" to control pain was common, so older patients often associate morphine with dying and are afraid that taking morphine means they are near death. The best response is to educate the patient about the different medications, but patients should be provided alternative medications if they feel strongly about taking morphine because taking it might increase their stress.

87. D: CHEOPS (Children's Hospital of Eastern Ontario Pain Scale) is used for children 1-7 and based on scores of 6 different characteristics (crying, facial expression, verbalization, torso, upper extremities, lower extremities) with scores of 0-2, except for crying, which is scored 0-3. A score more than 4 indicates pain. FACES (Wong-Baker): Facial expression scale for children older than 7. CRIES: Assesses crying, requirement for O_2 or SaO_2 less than 95%, increased vital signs (blood pressure and heart rate), expression, and sleep to evaluate pain in neonates and infants 6 months and younger. The 0-10 pain intensity scale is used with adolescents and adults.

88. B: While it seems logical that soothing music, such as classical music or New Age music, may be the most calming and relaxing, patient preference is more important because people react very differently to music. Playing a patient's favorite music can be very comforting and may help patients focus attention away from their pain or their situation. Dimming the lights and providing a quiet environment for music therapy help to relax the patient as well.

89. D: Midazolam 0.5 to 6 mg per hour intravenously (IV) is used for terminal/palliative sedation for patients who are highly agitated and in severe, uncontrolled pain. Midazolam is a very short-acting benzodiazepine with action beginning within 5 minutes and peaking at 20 to 60 minutes. Propofol, another IV agent, is also used, with starting does of 0.25 mg/kg/hr. Terminal sedation is indicated for patients when other medications and therapies have been unable to control their refractory symptoms.

90. D: Naloxone is a reversal agent (opiate antagonist) used for opioid narcotics, such as morphine. Patients must be monitored for hypertension and pulmonary edema after administration, and because the half-life is only approximately 20 minutes, repeat doses may be needed. Flumazenil is a reversal agent for benzodiazepines. N-acetylcysteine is a reversal agent for acetaminophen. Neostigmine is a reversal agent for nondepolarizing muscle relaxants. Reversal agents should always be available when patients are receiving high doses of opioids or benzodiazepines.

91. C: Ondansetron: Indicated for chemotherapy- and abdominal radiation–induced nausea and vomiting. It works well for both geriatric and pediatric patients. Dexamethasone may be given concurrently to potentiate effects. Haloperidol: Indicated for opioid-induced nausea as well as chemical- and mechanical-induced nausea, but can result in dyskinesia, although adverse effects are lessened with low doses. Scopolamine: Indicated for nausea and vomiting associated with intestinal obstruction, peritoneal irritation, and increased intracranial pressure. Dronabinol: Used as a second-line antiemetic, but more effective in young adults.

92. D: Corticosteroids, such as prednisone or dexamethasone, are used as adjuvant analgesics to relieve pain associated with spinal cord compression, cerebral edema, and bone pain, as well as visceral and neuropathic pain. Corticosteroids have anti-inflammatory effects that reduce swelling and inflammation. Prednisone may be given in doses of 15 to 30 mg three to four times daily. Dexamethasone is less likely to result in Cushing syndrome than prednisone. Dexamethasone may be given orally at 2 to 20 mg/day or IV (up to 100 mg bolus) for severe pain crisis.

93. A: Eutectic Mixture of Local Anesthetics (EMLA) cream provides good pain control. The skin is first cleansed and then the cream is applied thickly (1/4 inch), extending about 1/2 inch past the port to the peri-port tissue. The cream is then covered with plastic wrap, which is secured and left in place for about 20 minutes. The wrapped time may be extended to 45-60 minutes if necessary to completely numb the tissue. The tissue should remain numb for about 1 hour after the plastic wrap is removed, allowing time for the IV needle to be inserted and treatment begun.

94. C: With administration of ketamine, opioid dosage should be reduced by 50% because ketamine is a very strong analgesic at low doses. However, ketamine often causes hallucinations or nightmares, so lorazepam or diazepam (and sometimes haloperidol) is usually given as well, especially with moribund patients who may not be able to indicate that they are having hallucinations. Some people also have increased secretions and may need to receive an anticholinergic, such as glycopyrrolate or scopolamine, as well.

95. C: Physical dependence: Abrupt cessation of a drug and decrease in blood serum levels leads to withdrawal symptoms, which may vary depending on the type of drug. Addiction is a neurobiological disorder that includes lack of control over drug use, compulsive use of drugs, and continued craving for drugs despite negative effects. Tolerance is an adaptation in which a drug's effect diminishes over time so that an increased dose is needed to achieve the same effect. Pseudoaddiction is the mistaken belief that someone who is seeking drugs for pain is instead suffering from addiction.

96. A: Fentanyl patches may cause skin irritation, so it is important to rotate sites when reapplying the patches. Some patients find that spraying the skin with a steroid used for inhalation therapy prevents the skin reaction. The spray dries and does not leave residue that interferes with adherence or absorption. Powders, creams, ointments, and skin barriers cannot be used under the patches. If irritation persists, then patients may need to change to another form of analgesic.

97. B: Morphine 10 mg is equianalgesic to hydromorphone 1.5 mg. Hydromorphone (Dilaudid) is a hydrogenated ketone derivative of morphine. It is more highly lipid soluble than morphine and crosses the blood-brain barrier more readily, so it is faster acting than morphine and stronger (about 8 times). It has potent antitussive qualities. It produces less histamine release, nausea, and vomiting than morphine, so it is a good alternative if patients have an allergic response to morphine.

98. C: Complementary therapies are used in conjunction with conventional medical treatments, usually to help reduce pain, nausea, and anxiety, and to improve the quality of life. Complementary therapies encompass a wide variety of therapies, including aromatherapy, music therapy, acupuncture, massage, yoga, biofeedback, and hypnosis. Alternative therapies, on the other hand, are used in place of conventional medical treatments, usually to the patient's detriment. Alternative therapies include cancer-cure diets, oxygen therapy, and biomagnetic therapy, none of which have been demonstrated to actually work.

99. B: People who practice homeopathy believe that healing must occur from the inside and that they can use small doses of plants or minerals to promote healing by causing similar symptoms to the ones being treated ("like cures like"). Homeopathy prescribes specific substances for different diseases, depending on the patient's physical and emotional condition. The treatment usually does not include active ingredients found in medications, so the treatments rarely interfere with other medical treatment, although some people choose to use homeopathic treatment rather than traditional medication, and this can put the patient at risk.

100. A: Asian cultures tend to value stoicism, so Asian patients may not express pain with moaning or complaints, so the nurse cannot always use behavior as a guide when assessing a patient's degree of pain. Northern Europeans also tend to be fairly stoic. Hispanic, Middle Eastern, and southern European/Mediterranean cultures tend to be more expressive and their behavior may indicate pain is more severe than it actually is. While generalizations about culture may hold true for a culture as a whole, it is important to remember that they cannot necessarily be applied to any one individual in that culture.

101. A: This type of breakthrough pain is end-of-dose failure because the medication has peaked and the blood level is decreasing. A pain diary can help to establish the pattern of end-of-dose failure. The best solution is to either increase the dosage, usually by 25% to 50%, or to change the patch more frequently, such as every 48 hours. Increasing the use of oral opioids for the last 24 hours is not a good solution because the patient's pain is not being adequately controlled.

102. C: Incident pain follows a predictable pattern in that it occurs repeatedly with the same activity; therefore, the best solution is for the patient to take a rapid-onset, short-acting analgesic before attending the meeting. The pain medication can be titrated based on the patient's experience until the patient can carry out the activity with relative comfort. Oral transmucosal fentanyl citrate (OTFC) is often used for incident pain because the patient can take the medication easily and it works rapidly.

103. B: An abrupt change in behavior in a patient with end-stage dementia often means the patient is experiencing discomfort of some kind, so the nurse's initial intervention should be to try to determine the cause of discomfort, which may be related to constrictive clothing, pain, constipation, urinary retention, or urinary infection. Chemical restraints should be avoided, but a mild analgesic, such as acetaminophen, may be administered, and patients may benefit from a quiet environment with less stimulation if no cause for discomfort is identified.

104. A: SIADH is related to hypersecretion of the posterior pituitary gland, causing the kidneys to reabsorb fluids, resulting in fluid retention and a decrease in sodium levels (dilutional hyponatremia) but with production of only concentrated urine. SIADH may result from central nervous systems disorders, such as brain trauma, surgery, or tumors, as well as tumors of various organs, pneumothorax, acute pneumonia, other lung disorders, and some medications. Symptoms include the following:
anorexia with nausea and vomiting
irritability
stomach cramps
alterations of personality
increasing neurological dysfunction, including stupor and seizures, related to progressive sodium depletion.

105. C: As soon as possible after a patient dies, the nurse should gently apply downward pressure on the eyelids to close them. *Rigor mortis* begins in small muscles, so the eyes may remain open if the eyelids are not closed soon after death. This can be disconcerting to family members. The mouth should not be tied closed, although a rolled towel may be placed under the chin to attempt to close the mouth. Dentures should not be placed in the mouth, as loose dentures can easily be lost. Dentures should be sent to the funeral home with the deceased.

106. B: It is important to ask patients directly about their needs, and patients may be more willing to discuss needs if the nurse acknowledges directly that a patient has received bad news, rather than talking around the subject or asking open-ended questions, such as "Do you need anything?" The nurse should stay focused on the patients and their needs and feelings rather than personal feelings, "I feel terrible for you." The nurse can also offer suggestions, "Some patients have needed…"

107. D: Independent decision-making is not a primary benefit of working with an interdisciplinary team because important decisions should be reached by group consensus, although even in groups, some independent decisions, such as when a patient requires pain medication, are reached by an individual. Working in an interdisciplinary group allows people to learn from each other because members have different expertise, and this aids in problem-solving. Additionally, the group can serve as a support system for the members.

108. B: Most patients are able to easily tolerate infusion of subcutaneous fluids per hypodermoclysis at the rate of 100 mL/hr. If this absorbs readily, then the rate may be increased. Up to about 1500 mL can usually be instilled at one site. Hypodermoclysis is usually administered to tissue of the abdomen or anterior or lateral thighs. Patients should be monitored for pain. Complications can include infection, tissue sloughing with over-infusion, third spacing, and local irritation and bleeding.

109. D: Dehydration at the end of life results in effects on all systems, including the pulmonary system. As airways dry, secretions lessen, and the ability to cough is reduced. The death rattle also begins to lessen. Patients exhibit less wheezing and dyspnea. Rehydration, on the other hand, makes suctioning easier and allows for more productive cough, although as patients weaken, their ability to cough decreases and fluids begin to pool, resulting in the death rattle.

110. C: A right hemisphere stroke usually does not interfere with language skills, so the nurse should speak normally. A right hemisphere stroke results in left paralysis or paresis and a left visual field deficit that may cause spatial and perceptual disturbances, so patients may have difficulty judging distance. Fine motor skills may be impacted, resulting in trouble dressing or handling tools. People may become impulsive and exhibit poor judgment, often denying impairment. Left-sided neglect (lack of perception of things on the left side) may occur. Depression is common as well as short-term memory loss and difficulty following directions.

111. A: Oral phase: Patient has difficulty chewing and swallowing and tends to drool liquids and food and has food remaining in the mouth after finishing the meal. Pharyngeal phase: Patient chokes while swallowing and often regurgitates food into the nose during the meal or immediately afterward. Breath sounds and voice may be gurgling after eating because of incomplete swallowing, and patients may feel as though food is "caught in the throat." Esophageal phase: Patient has reflux and regurgitates food frequently after eating and has difficulty swallowing solid foods. Patient may complain of difficulty swallowing but rarely coughs or chokes, and may feel as though food is caught in the chest.

112. B: Variant angina (also known as Prinzmetal angina) results from spasms of the coronary arteries and can be associated with or without atherosclerotic plaques; it is often related to smoking, alcohol, or illicit stimulants. ST-segment elevation usually occurs with variant angina. Variant angina frequently occurs cyclically at the same time each day and often while the person is at rest. Nitroglycerine or calcium channel blockers are used for treatment, but beta-blockers should be avoided.

113. A: Virchow's triad comprises common risk factors for acute venous thromboembolism: blood stasis, injury to endothelium, and hypercoagulability. Some patients may be initially asymptomatic, but symptoms may include aching or throbbing pain, positive Homan's sign (pain in calf when foot is dorsiflexed), erythema and edema, dilation of vessels, and cyanosis.

114. D: Both type 1 and type 2 diabetes can result in macrovascular (atherosclerotic plaques) and microvascular (capillary) damage:
Microvascular: Retinopathy can lead to blindness; neuropathy causes nerve damage that can lead to diabetic gastroparesis, bladder dysfunction, diabetic foot ulcers, pain, and loss of sensation. Nephropathy can lead to chronic renal failure and the need for dialysis.
Macrovascular: Atherosclerosis of the coronary and cerebral arteries and peripheral arteries can result in peripheral vascular disease, stroke, and myocardial infarction.

115. D: Because of the severe discomfort and difficulty breathing associated with tense ascites, paracentesis is frequently used to relieve symptoms. However, the fluid recurs, so it is important to educate the patient and family about the importance of restricting fluids and sodium intake. No more than 6 L of fluid should be removed at one time with paracentesis. Spironolactone is the diuretic of choice, but furosemide may also be used to initiate diuresis. Patients should be advised to suck on hard candy or ice cubes to help alleviate thirst.

116. D: A patient on a mechanically altered diet needs foods that are finely ground or chopped and that require minimal chewing but can easily form an adequate cohesive bolus because the patient has limitations in chewing and poor tongue control. These foods include pasta, cottage cheese, moistened ground meats, and soft scrambled eggs. Fruits should be cooked or canned with seeds and skin removed. Foods to avoid include raw or dried fruits and vegetables, nuts, chips (taco, potato), hard rolls, waffles, and any meat that requires extensive chewing.

117. B: Xerostomia (dry mouth) is a common problem with cancer patients and may result from medications, chemotherapy, radiation, and disease processes. Pilocarpine is a nonselective muscarinic that increases saliva production, but it may result in increased perspiration, nausea, flushing, and cramping. Management includes treating cause (if possible), reviewing medications, stimulating flow of saliva, and using saliva substitutes; however, these remedies may provide only partial relief. Acupuncture treatments have increased saliva production for some patients.

118. A: Most cases of persistent hiccoughs result from gastric distention, as in this case. The initial medication treatment should be to reduce gastric distention with simethicone (15 to 30 mL by mouth every 4 hours) or metoclopramide (10 to 20 mg by mouth or intravenously every 4 to 6 hours). Other nonpharmacologic approaches to relieving gastric distention include fasting or induced vomiting, gastric lavage, and insertion of a nasogastric tube for decompression. Other treatments for hiccoughs include muscle relaxants, corticosteroids, dopamine agonists, anticonvulsants, calcium channel blockers, and SSRIs.

- 120 -

119. D: Stimulant laxatives are recommended for opioid-related constipation in the chronically ill patient. A typical protocol begins with Senokot-S (standardized senna concentrate and docusate sodium) 2 tablets at bedtime with dosage increased if no bowel movement. Bulk laxatives are used for mild constipation and may worsen constipation if fluid intake is inadequate. Osmotic laxatives are also useful for opioid-related constipation, but many patients are unable to tolerate the sweet taste or the resulting gas and distention. Saline laxatives can cause severe cramping and pain and should be used as a last resort for chronically ill patients.

120. D: Most opioids can cause pruritus, but morphine, which causes more histamine release, is more likely to cause pruritus than other opioids such as fentanyl, codeine, and oxymorphone. If itching is mild, an antihistamine given concurrently may control itching, but in some cases discontinuing the morphine and switching to another drug or rotating between morphine and another drug may be necessary. Application of cold may help relieve itching to a localized area, but heat often increases itching. Topical antipruritics, such as hydrocortisone, may relieve itching but are not practical if itching is generalized.

121. A: Of the primary breast and prostate cancers that metastasize, two-thirds metastasize first to bone. About one-third of metastasizing primary lung, thyroid, and kidney cancers metastasize to bone. If the metastasizing cancer activates osteoblasts, lytic lesions (holes) form in the bones, weakening the bones and increasing risk of fracture. If the metastasizing cancer activates osteoblasts, blastic lesions cause sclerosis of the bones, which hardens them, so blastic lesions are not as likely to cause pathological fractures as lytic lesions.

122. C: Because of headaches and altered consciousness associated with increased intracranial pressure, the best position is with the head of the bed raised to 30 to 45 degrees. The head and neck should be maintained in neutral position with bolsters to facilitate jugular venous return because this may help to decrease the intracranial pressure. The patient should be tilted from side to side, keeping head in neutral position, to prevent pressure sores, and good skin care should be provided.

123. D: Studies show that over a quarter of the patients with cancer experience both fatigue and depression, with each condition exacerbating the other. Other factors that may increase fatigue include anemia, especially common with patients who have received chemotherapy, have experienced bleeding, and have nutritional deficits. Fatigue may also be related to sleep disorders, especially in older adults. Other contributing factors include infection, hormonal imbalances, and electrolyte imbalances. Patients may need to modify their activities and include more rest time.

124. C: There is little that has been able to reverse anorexia/cachexia when people are in advanced stages of disease, and telling a patient she must eat to live will only add to her stress. However, some strategies can help to slow the process. Patients often do better eating small amounts every hour or two and supplementing their diet with nutritional drinks, such as Ensure, to increase calories and nutrients. The nurse should explore dietary preferences with the patient, trying to find foods that the patient feels like eating; however, this can prove challenging and may vary from day to day.

125. A: Extended-release formulas of tolterodine and oxybutynin cause mild to moderate mouth dryness, while older preparations tend to cause moderate to severe mouth dryness. For a patient who is having difficulty eating, changing medications and taking the medication at bedtime rather than in the morning can reduce mouth dryness. The patient should also be taught behavioral remedies, such as urge suppression techniques, and be advised to urinate on a timed schedule because medications alone are not always sufficient.

126. C: While the Medicare Hospice Benefit does not cover curative care for the patient's terminal illness, it does cover curative care for incidental conditions such as an infection or injuries and treatment to control pain and symptoms. Hospice does not cover the costs of extended live-in 24-hour care and requires that hospice services be provided by Medicare-approved hospice providers. The hospice benefit also does not cover ambulance and emergency department services unless arranged for by the hospice provider.

127. B: While individual needs vary, many individuals under hospice care find long periods of time alone difficult, so a friendly visitors program in which the same volunteer comes to the patient's home can be invaluable. Friendly visitors usually make visits on a regular schedule, often weekly, in addition to contacting the patient by telephone and in some cases arranging for outings, such as a taking the patient who is able for a drive. Volunteers in hospice programs should undergo screening and training before visiting patients.

128. A: The best solution is "Let's make a list of questions to give the doctor," because this is a practical solution that responds directly to the patient's concerns. Many hospice patients suffer from fatigue and the thought of writing out a list of questions on their own may seem daunting. In the process of exploring questions, the nurse may find some that he or she can respond to, and this can lead to worthwhile discussions because some questions may not require physician input.

129. B: With lower-extremity lymphedema, there is an increased risk of fungal infection of the toes, so antifungal powder should be applied routinely and the patient advised to wear cotton socks and breathable shoes (such as canvas). Signs of fungal infection include redness, itching, and peeling of skin. Antibiotics are given for infections, which are common complications because of stasis and accumulated debris in tissues. Antibiotics may be given prophylactically if patients have repeated infections. Oral antifungal agents are not generally used prophylactically.

130. C: High-air-loss support surfaces promote the evaporation of moisture by passing air over the skin. High-air-loss (air-fluidized) support surfaces also provide an increased support area and reduced accumulation of heat. They reduce pressure and shear. The typical standard hospital bed mattress has none of these qualities. The common foam support surface provides little more protection than the mattress.

131. B: Hydrocolloids are probably the best choice because they provide absorption for small to medium amounts of exudate and provide a warm, moist environment for healing. They can be left in place for 2 to 5 days, but they do pose an increased risk of anaerobic infection. Gauze dressings should not be applied directly to an open wound because they will adhere and damage the tissue. Semi-permeable film is appropriate for dry wounds. Alginate dressings are used for wounds with large amounts of dressing because of their absorptive properties.

132. C: Patients may have insurance coverage for direct medical costs, such as medications, treatments, physician's visits, durable medical equipment, and emergency services. Direct nonmedical costs are those that result from the illness, such as lost income from missed employment, transportation costs, and caregiver costs. These direct nonmedical costs are usually not covered by insurance and may pose a severe financial hardship on patients and their families, so these costs need to be considered when people are planning care.

133. C: These symptoms are consistent with pleural effusion, with increasing dyspnea as the most common symptom. As the pleural fluid builds, the pressure may cause the lung to collapse. Patients

often exhibit a dry, nonproductive cough and pain and heaviness in the chest. If the pleural effusion is extensive, it may result in a mediastinal shift. Thoracentesis may relieve symptoms, but fluid usually accumulates again within a few days. Other treatment options include sclerotherapy, pleuroperitoneal shunt, pleurectomy, indwelling catheters, and subcutaneous access ports.

134. A: Poorly controlled symptoms, such as pain and nausea, are the most likely to have a negative impact on a patient's ability to maintain a feeling of hope at the end of life, so managing symptoms should be the first priority of care. The nurse should ask patients directly how well they are controlling their symptoms and how this is affecting their sense of hope. The nurse should also ask the patient about who provides support—emotional, physical, and spiritual—and methods they use to handle difficult situations.

135. C: Disenfranchised grief: Grief expressed in secret because it is not socially sanctioned, such as that of a lover, unacknowledged illegitimate child, or mistress. The person may not be able to see the dying person or attend memorial services or funerals. Unresolved grief: Grief that persists because the person is unable to work through the grief to find resolution. Complicated grief: Grief that persists more than 1 year and intrudes on thoughts and abilities to function. Uncomplicated grief: Grief that results in an emotional reaction and then a period of recovery.

136. D: The death of a parent is almost always devastating to a child, and a parent's instinct is often to protect and shield the child from the reality of the illness, but this can result in complicated grief and anger. Children need to be involved in care to the level of their ability. For example, a child can do light tasks, such as bringing water or books to the parent, and provide comfort measures, such as reading or singing to the parent, holding the parent's hand, and even just sitting with the parent. Children are less frightened if people are honest with them and if they feel useful and needed.

137. D: According to the Clinical Practice Guidelines of the National Consensus Project, bereavement and follow-up services must be offered to family members after a patient's death for a minimum of 12 months. Grief and bereavement services should be available and offered by trained staff to both the patient and family members throughout the period of illness. Families should be apprised of services with information that is appropriate for their culture and linguistic abilities.

138. C: Under Quality Assurance and Performance Improvement (QAPI), Element 4, performance improvement projects must be identified within the facility and can apply to one area or department or to the entire facility, depending on the breadth of the project. The goal is a continuing effort to identify problems and improve services. QAPI includes 5 elements:
1. Designs and Scope.
2. Governance and Leadership.
3. Feedback, Data Systems, and Monitoring.
4. Performance Improvement Projects (PIPs).
5. Systematic Analysis and Systemic Action.

139. B: This is clearly a professional boundary violation, even though these actions may appear caring. In fact, since a professional relationship exists between the patient and the nurse, there are liability issues if the nurse is visiting when off-duty, especially if the nurse is providing care and a problem arises. Additionally, the nurse is creating a relationship of dependency on the part of the patient and family, and seeking to fulfill personal needs by being overinvested in patients' lives.

140. D: The primary principle of palliative care is to focus on relieving suffering for the dying person. All aspects of care should be focused on that goal while attending to the medical, social,

psychological, and spiritual needs of the patient and family members. The nurse must serve as an advocate for the patient and family to help them gain access to needed services and care settings in order to receive excellent care at the end of life.

141. A: Patients with history of drug abuse are entitled to adequate pain control, but they must be assessed and evaluated carefully. Of special concern are patients who roll and smoke fentanyl patches because this releases a 3-day supply of the drug rapidly and can result in a life-threatening overdose. Patients with a history of drug abuse may have developed a tolerance to drugs, so taking medications before the scheduled time and asking for higher doses is not uncommon; however, some patients react in the opposite way and are fearful of taking pain medications.

142. C: Terminal sedation differs from physician-assisted suicide in that it is primarily intended to provide comfort and alleviate suffering, and the hastening of death that may occur is a secondary effect. The primary purpose of physician-assisted suicide is to bring about a patient's death (even though it is also intended to provide comfort and alleviate suffering). These are legal distinctions. In most states, physician-assisted suicide is illegal, but the US Supreme Court has upheld the rights of individuals to have terminal sedation to alleviate symptoms.

143. D: Patients should be medicated prior to extubation and have additional medications available to control symptoms. The medications that are most indicated to relieve a sense of breathlessness are opioids. Benzodiazepines are also usually administered to relieve anxiety. Oxygen is usually continued at about 21%. If family chooses to stay at the bedside while the patient is dying, the nurse should make sure that they can remain close to the patient and can encourage them to hold the person's hand or touch the patient.

144. C: Grade 3. National Cancer Institute Scale of Severity of Diarrhea:
Grade 0: Normal stools.
Grade 1: Two to three stools daily but essentially no other symptoms.
Grade 2: Four to six stools daily with stools at night and/or moderate abdominal cramping.
Grade 3: Seven to nine stool daily with fecal incontinence and/or severe abdominal cramping.
Grade 4: More than 10 stools daily with stools grossly bloody and/or fluid depletion results in need for parenteral support.

145. B: "Huffing" is an airway clearance technique to improve cough effectiveness so patients are better able to expectorate secretions. The patient is instructed to lie on his or her side while holding a pillow against the abdomen for support. The patient takes a deep breath and then "huffs" or breathes out sharply three or four times in bursts with the mouth open. This type of coughing is less tiring than a forceful cough and may help to clear mucus for all patients with cough.

146. A: Because bacterial colonization of the necrotic wound results in a foul odor, the most effective treatment is usually application of a metronidazole topical solution (0.5% to 1%) to the wound surface. It can also be used to irrigate the wound and saturate dressings. Metronidazole topical gel (0.75%) is also available and applied in a thin film to the wound. Yogurt has been applied to necrotic wounds with some success, and skin cleansers and charcoal dressings are also helpful.

147. D: Cost minimization: Based on the assumption that two treatments are equal in effectiveness, so the least expensive option should be utilized. Cost effectiveness: Compares treatments and assigns dollar value to each year of life gained by a treatment. Cost utility: Similar to cost-effectiveness but estimates the value in quality of life. Cost benefit: Evaluates treatments in terms of monetary value of life; assigning a dollar value to life is difficult, so this approach is seldom used.

148. A: The three primary aspects of evidence-based practice are clinical expertise, best available research, and patient values. These three aspects guide decision-making in relation to patient care in order to promote optimal outcomes. Clinical expertise includes both education and experience. The best available research is based on research conducted using scientific methodology and often reported on in juried publications and at conferences. Patient values and wishes are important components of evidence-based practice.

149. C: Fractionated external-beam radiation therapy is the primary treatment for spinal cord compression because it inhibits the growth of tumor and is often able to restore and preserve neurological function. After treatment, most patients will retain the ability to ambulate; of those already paraparetic and unable to walk, over a third will regain this ability, although only about 5% of patients with paraplegia progress to the point that they can walk again. Dexamethasone is the corticosteroid of choice. Decompressive surgery is an option for some patients.

150. B: The Agency for Healthcare Research and Quality recommends use of the ABCDE method for assessing and managing pain:
A. Asking patient about the extent of pain and assessing systematically.
B. Believing that the degree of pain the patient reports is accurate.
C. Choosing the appropriate method of pain control for the patient and circumstances.
D. Delivering pain interventions appropriately and in a timely, logical manner.
E. Empowering patients and family by helping them to have control of the course of treatment.

Secret Key #1 - Time is Your Greatest Enemy

Pace Yourself

Wear a watch. At the beginning of the test, check the time (or start a chronometer on your watch to count the minutes), and check the time after every few questions to make sure you are "on schedule."

If you are forced to speed up, do it efficiently. Usually one or more answer choices can be eliminated without too much difficulty. Above all, don't panic. Don't speed up and just begin guessing at random choices. By pacing yourself, and continually monitoring your progress against your watch, you will always know exactly how far ahead or behind you are with your available time. If you find that you are one minute behind on the test, don't skip one question without spending any time on it, just to catch back up. Take 15 fewer seconds on the next four questions, and after four questions you'll have caught back up. Once you catch back up, you can continue working each problem at your normal pace.

Furthermore, don't dwell on the problems that you were rushed on. If a problem was taking up too much time and you made a hurried guess, it must be difficult. The difficult questions are the ones you are most likely to miss anyway, so it isn't a big loss. It is better to end with more time than you need than to run out of time.

Lastly, sometimes it is beneficial to slow down if you are constantly getting ahead of time. You are always more likely to catch a careless mistake by working more slowly than quickly, and among very high-scoring test takers (those who are likely to have lots of time left over), careless errors affect the score more than mastery of material.

Secret Key #2 - Guessing is not Guesswork

You probably know that guessing is a good idea - unlike other standardized tests, there is no penalty for getting a wrong answer. Even if you have no idea about a question, you still have a 20-25% chance of getting it right.

Most test takers do not understand the impact that proper guessing can have on their score. Unless you score extremely high, guessing will significantly contribute to your final score.

Monkeys Take the Test

What most test takers don't realize is that to insure that 20-25% chance, you have to guess randomly. If you put 20 monkeys in a room to take this test, assuming they answered once per question and behaved themselves, on average they would get 20-25% of the questions correct. Put 20 test takers in the room, and the average will be much lower among guessed questions. Why?

1. The test writers intentionally writes deceptive answer choices that "look" right. A test taker has no idea about a question, so picks the "best looking" answer, which is often wrong. The monkey has no idea what looks good and what doesn't, so will consistently be lucky about 20-25% of the time.
2. Test takers will eliminate answer choices from the guessing pool based on a hunch or intuition. Simple but correct answers often get excluded, leaving a 0% chance of being correct. The monkey has no clue, and often gets lucky with the best choice.

This is why the process of elimination endorsed by most test courses is flawed and detrimental to your performance- test takers don't guess, they make an ignorant stab in the dark that is usually worse than random.

$5 Challenge

Let me introduce one of the most valuable ideas of this course- the $5 challenge:
You only mark your "best guess" if you are willing to bet $5 on it.
You only eliminate choices from guessing if you are willing to bet $5 on it.

Why $5? Five dollars is an amount of money that is small yet not insignificant, and can really add up fast (20 questions could cost you $100). Likewise, each answer choice on one question of the test will have a small impact on your overall score, but it can really add up to a lot of points in the end.

The process of elimination IS valuable. The following shows your chance of guessing it right:

If you eliminate wrong answer choices until only this many answer choices remain:	Chance of getting it correct:
1	100%
2	50%
3	33%

However, if you accidentally eliminate the right answer or go on a hunch for an incorrect answer, your chances drop dramatically: to 0%. By guessing among all the answer choices, you are GUARANTEED to have a shot at the right answer.

That's why the $5 test is so valuable- if you give up the advantage and safety of a pure guess, it had better be worth the risk.

What we still haven't covered is how to be sure that whatever guess you make is truly random. Here's the easiest way:

Always pick the first answer choice among those remaining.

Such a technique means that you have decided, **before you see a single test question**, exactly how you are going to guess- and since the order of choices tells you nothing about which one is correct, this guessing technique is perfectly random.

This section is not meant to scare you away from making educated guesses or eliminating choices- you just need to define when a choice is worth eliminating. The $5 test, along with a pre-defined random guessing strategy, is the best way to make sure you reap all of the benefits of guessing.

Secret Key #3 - Practice Smarter, Not Harder

Many test takers delay the test preparation process because they dread the awful amounts of practice time they think necessary to succeed on the test. We have refined an effective method that will take you only a fraction of the time.

There are a number of "obstacles" in your way to succeed. Among these are answering questions, finishing in time, and mastering test-taking strategies. All must be executed on the day of the test at peak performance, or your score will suffer. The test is a mental marathon that has a large impact on your future.

Just like a marathon runner, it is important to work your way up to the full challenge. So first you just worry about questions, and then time, and finally strategy:

Success Strategy

1. Find a good source for practice tests.
2. If you are willing to make a larger time investment, consider using more than one study guide- often the different approaches of multiple authors will help you "get" difficult concepts.
3. Take a practice test with no time constraints, with all study helps "open book." Take your time with questions and focus on applying strategies.
4. Take a practice test with time constraints, with all guides "open book."
5. Take a final practice test with no open material and time limits

If you have time to take more practice tests, just repeat step 5. By gradually exposing yourself to the full rigors of the test environment, you will condition your mind to the stress of test day and maximize your success.

Secret Key #4 - Prepare, Don't Procrastinate

Let me state an obvious fact: if you take the test three times, you will get three different scores. This is due to the way you feel on test day, the level of preparedness you have, and, despite the test writers' claims to the contrary, some tests WILL be easier for you than others.

Since your future depends so much on your score, you should maximize your chances of success. In order to maximize the likelihood of success, you've got to prepare in advance. This means taking practice tests and spending time learning the information and test taking strategies you will need to succeed.

Never take the test as a "practice" test, expecting that you can just take it again if you need to. Feel free to take sample tests on your own, but when you go to take the official test, be prepared, be focused, and do your best the first time!

Secret Key #5 - Test Yourself

Everyone knows that time is money. There is no need to spend too much of your time or too little of your time preparing for the test. You should only spend as much of your precious time preparing as is necessary for you to get the score you need.

Once you have taken a practice test under real conditions of time constraints, then you will know if you are ready for the test or not.

If you have scored extremely high the first time that you take the practice test, then there is not much point in spending countless hours studying. You are already there.

Benchmark your abilities by retaking practice tests and seeing how much you have improved. Once you score high enough to guarantee success, then you are ready.

If you have scored well below where you need, then knuckle down and begin studying in earnest. Check your improvement regularly through the use of practice tests under real conditions. Above all, don't worry, panic, or give up. The key is perseverance!

Then, when you go to take the test, remain confident and remember how well you did on the practice tests. If you can score high enough on a practice test, then you can do the same on the real thing.

General Strategies

The most important thing you can do is to ignore your fears and jump into the test immediately- do not be overwhelmed by any strange-sounding terms. You have to jump into the test like jumping into a pool- all at once is the easiest way.

Make Predictions

As you read and understand the question, try to guess what the answer will be. Remember that several of the answer choices are wrong, and once you begin reading them, your mind will immediately become cluttered with answer choices designed to throw you off. Your mind is typically the most focused immediately after you have read the question and digested its contents. If you can, try to predict what the correct answer will be. You may be surprised at what you can predict.

Quickly scan the choices and see if your prediction is in the listed answer choices. If it is, then you can be quite confident that you have the right answer. It still won't hurt to check the other answer choices, but most of the time, you've got it!

Answer the Question

It may seem obvious to only pick answer choices that answer the question, but the test writers can create some excellent answer choices that are wrong. Don't pick an answer just because it sounds right, or you believe it to be true. It MUST answer the question. Once you've made your selection, always go back and check it against the question and make sure that you didn't misread the question, and the answer choice does answer the question posed.

Benchmark

After you read the first answer choice, decide if you think it sounds correct or not. If it doesn't, move on to the next answer choice. If it does, mentally mark that answer choice. This doesn't mean that you've definitely selected it as your answer choice, it just means that it's the best you've seen thus far. Go ahead and read the next choice. If the next choice is worse than the one you've already selected, keep going to the next answer choice. If the next choice is better than the choice you've already selected, mentally mark the new answer choice as your best guess.

The first answer choice that you select becomes your standard. Every other answer choice must be benchmarked against that standard. That choice is correct until proven otherwise by another answer choice beating it out. Once you've decided that no other answer choice seems as good, do one final check to ensure that your answer choice answers the question posed.

Valid Information

Don't discount any of the information provided in the question. Every piece of information may be necessary to determine the correct answer. None of the information in the question is there to throw you off (while the answer choices will certainly have information to throw you off). If two seemingly unrelated topics are discussed, don't ignore either. You can be confident there is a relationship, or it wouldn't be included in the question, and you are probably going to have to determine what is that relationship to find the answer.

Avoid "Fact Traps"

Don't get distracted by a choice that is factually true. Your search is for the answer that answers the question. Stay focused and don't fall for an answer that is true but incorrect. Always go back to the question and make sure you're choosing an answer that actually answers the question and is not just a true statement. An answer can be factually correct, but it MUST answer the question asked. Additionally, two answers can both be seemingly correct, so be sure to read all of the answer choices, and make sure that you get the one that BEST answers the question.

Milk the Question

Some of the questions may throw you completely off. They might deal with a subject you have not been exposed to, or one that you haven't reviewed in years. While your lack of knowledge about the subject will be a hindrance, the question itself can give you many clues that will help you find the correct answer. Read the question carefully and look for clues. Watch particularly for adjectives and nouns describing difficult terms or words that you don't recognize. Regardless of if you completely understand a word or not, replacing it with a synonym either provided or one you more familiar with may help you to understand what the questions are asking. Rather than wracking your mind about specific detailed information concerning a difficult term or word, try to use mental substitutes that are easier to understand.

The Trap of Familiarity

Don't just choose a word because you recognize it. On difficult questions, you may not recognize a number of words in the answer choices. The test writers don't put "make-believe" words on the test; so don't think that just because you only recognize all the words in one answer choice means that answer choice must be correct. If you only recognize words in one answer choice, then focus on that one. Is it correct? Try your best to determine if it is correct. If it is, that is great, but if it doesn't, eliminate it. Each word and answer choice you eliminate increases your chances of getting the question correct, even if you then have to guess among the unfamiliar choices.

Eliminate Answers

Eliminate choices as soon as you realize they are wrong. But be careful! Make sure you consider all of the possible answer choices. Just because one appears right, doesn't mean that the next one won't be even better! The test writers will usually put more than one good answer choice for every question, so read all of them. Don't worry if you are stuck between two that seem right. By getting down to just two remaining possible choices, your odds are now 50/50. Rather than wasting too much time, play the odds. You are guessing, but guessing wisely, because you've been able to knock out some of the answer choices that you know are wrong. If you are eliminating choices and realize that the last answer choice you are left with is also obviously wrong, don't panic. Start over and consider each choice again. There may easily be something that you missed the first time and will realize on the second pass.

Tough Questions

If you are stumped on a problem or it appears too hard or too difficult, don't waste time. Move on! Remember though, if you can quickly check for obviously incorrect answer choices, your chances of guessing correctly are greatly improved. Before you completely give up, at least try to knock out a couple of possible answers. Eliminate what you can and then guess at the remaining answer choices before moving on.

Brainstorm

If you get stuck on a difficult question, spend a few seconds quickly brainstorming. Run through the complete list of possible answer choices. Look at each choice and ask yourself, "Could this answer the question satisfactorily?" Go through each answer choice and consider it independently of the other. By systematically going through all possibilities, you may find something that you would otherwise overlook. Remember that when you get stuck, it's important to try to keep moving.

Read Carefully

Understand the problem. Read the question and answer choices carefully. Don't miss the question because you misread the terms. You have plenty of time to read each question thoroughly and make sure you understand what is being asked. Yet a happy medium must be attained, so don't waste too much time. You must read carefully, but efficiently.

Face Value

When in doubt, use common sense. Always accept the situation in the problem at face value. Don't read too much into it. These problems will not require you to make huge leaps of logic. The test writers aren't trying to throw you off with a cheap trick. If you have to go beyond creativity and make a leap of logic in order to have an answer choice answer the question, then you should look at the other answer choices. Don't overcomplicate the problem by creating theoretical relationships or explanations that will warp time or space. These are normal problems rooted in reality. It's just that the applicable relationship or explanation may not be readily apparent and you have to figure things out. Use your common sense to interpret anything that isn't clear.

Prefixes

If you're having trouble with a word in the question or answer choices, try dissecting it. Take advantage of every clue that the word might include. Prefixes and suffixes can be a huge help. Usually they allow you to determine a basic meaning. Pre- means before, post- means after, pro - is positive, de- is negative. From these prefixes and suffixes, you can get an idea of the general meaning of the word and try to put it into context. Beware though of any traps. Just because con is the opposite of pro, doesn't necessarily mean congress is the opposite of progress!

Hedge Phrases

Watch out for critical "hedge" phrases, such as likely, may, can, will often, sometimes, often, almost, mostly, usually, generally, rarely, sometimes. Question writers insert these hedge phrases to cover every possibility. Often an answer choice will be wrong simply because it leaves no room for exception. Avoid answer choices that have definitive words like "exactly," and "always".

Switchback Words

Stay alert for "switchbacks". These are the words and phrases frequently used to alert you to shifts in thought. The most common switchback word is "but". Others include although, however, nevertheless, on the other hand, even though, while, in spite of, despite, regardless of.

New Information

Correct answer choices will rarely have completely new information included. Answer choices typically are straightforward reflections of the material asked about and will directly relate to the question. If a new piece of information is included in an answer choice that doesn't even seem to relate to the topic being asked about, then that answer choice is likely incorrect. All of the information needed to answer the question is usually provided for you, and so you should not have to make guesses that are unsupported or choose answer choices that require unknown information that cannot be reasoned on its own.

Time Management

On technical questions, don't get lost on the technical terms. Don't spend too much time on any one question. If you don't know what a term means, then since you don't have a dictionary, odds are you aren't going to get much further. You should immediately recognize terms as whether or not you know them. If you don't, work with the other clues that you have, the other answer choices and terms provided, but don't waste too much time trying to figure out a difficult term.

Contextual Clues

Look for contextual clues. An answer can be right but not correct. The contextual clues will help you find the answer that is most right and is correct. Understand the context in which a phrase or statement is made. This will help you make important distinctions.

Don't Panic

Panicking will not answer any questions for you. Therefore, it isn't helpful. When you first see the question, if your mind goes blank, take a deep breath. Force yourself to mechanically go through the steps of solving the problem and using the strategies you've learned.

Pace Yourself

Don't get clock fever. It's easy to be overwhelmed when you're looking at a page full of questions, your mind is full of random thoughts and feeling confused, and the clock is ticking down faster than you would like. Calm down and maintain the pace that you have set for yourself. As long as you are on track by monitoring your pace, you are guaranteed to have enough time for yourself. When you get to the last few minutes of the test, it may seem like you won't have enough time left, but if you only have as many questions as you should have left at that point, then you're right on track!

Answer Selection

The best way to pick an answer choice is to eliminate all of those that are wrong, until only one is left and confirm that is the correct answer. Sometimes though, an answer choice may immediately look right. Be careful! Take a second to make sure that the other choices are not equally obvious. Don't make a hasty mistake. There are only two times that you should stop before checking other answers. First is when you are positive that the answer choice you have selected is correct. Second is when time is almost out and you have to make a quick guess!

Check Your Work

Since you will probably not know every term listed and the answer to every question, it is important that you get credit for the ones that you do know. Don't miss any questions through careless mistakes. If at all possible, try to take a second to look back over your answer selection and make sure you've selected the correct answer choice and haven't made a costly careless mistake (such as marking an answer choice that you didn't mean to mark). This quick double check should more than pay for itself in caught mistakes for the time it costs.

Beware of Directly Quoted Answers

Sometimes an answer choice will repeat word for word a portion of the question or reference section. However, beware of such exact duplication – it may be a trap! More than likely, the correct choice will paraphrase or summarize a point, rather than being exactly the same wording.

Slang

Scientific sounding answers are better than slang ones. An answer choice that begins "To compare the outcomes..." is much more likely to be correct than one that begins "Because some people insisted..."

Extreme Statements

Avoid wild answers that throw out highly controversial ideas that are proclaimed as established fact. An answer choice that states the "process should be used in certain situations, if..." is much more likely to be correct than one that states the "process should be discontinued completely." The first is a calm rational statement and doesn't even make a definitive, uncompromising stance, using a hedge word "if" to provide wiggle room, whereas the second choice is a radical idea and far more extreme.

Answer Choice Families

When you have two or more answer choices that are direct opposites or parallels, one of them is usually the correct answer. For instance, if one answer choice states "x increases" and another answer choice states "x decreases" or "y increases," then those two or three answer choices are very similar in construction and fall into the same family of answer choices. A family of answer choices is when two or three answer choices are very similar in construction, and yet often have a directly opposite meaning. Usually the correct answer choice will be in that family of answer choices. The "odd man out" or answer choice that doesn't seem to fit the parallel construction of the other answer choices is more likely to be incorrect.

Special Report: How to Overcome Test Anxiety

The very nature of tests caters to some level of anxiety, nervousness, or tension, just as we feel for any important event that occurs in our lives. A little bit of anxiety or nervousness can be a good thing. It helps us with motivation, and makes achievement just that much sweeter. However, too much anxiety can be a problem, especially if it hinders our ability to function and perform.

"Test anxiety," is the term that refers to the emotional reactions that some test-takers experience when faced with a test or exam. Having a fear of testing and exams is based upon a rational fear, since the test-taker's performance can shape the course of an academic career. Nevertheless, experiencing excessive fear of examinations will only interfere with the test-taker's ability to perform and chance to be successful.

There are a large variety of causes that can contribute to the development and sensation of test anxiety. These include, but are not limited to, lack of preparation and worrying about issues surrounding the test.

Lack of Preparation

Lack of preparation can be identified by the following behaviors or situations:

Not scheduling enough time to study, and therefore cramming the night before the test or exam
Managing time poorly, to create the sensation that there is not enough time to do everything
Failing to organize the text information in advance, so that the study material consists of the entire text and not simply the pertinent information
Poor overall studying habits

Worrying, on the other hand, can be related to both the test taker, or many other factors around him/her that will be affected by the results of the test. These include worrying about:

Previous performances on similar exams, or exams in general
How friends and other students are achieving
The negative consequences that will result from a poor grade or failure

There are three primary elements to test anxiety. Physical components, which involve the same typical bodily reactions as those to acute anxiety (to be discussed below). Emotional factors have to do with fear or panic. Mental or cognitive issues concerning attention spans and memory abilities.

Physical Signals

There are many different symptoms of test anxiety, and these are not limited to mental and emotional strain. Frequently there are a range of physical signals that will let a test taker know that he/she is suffering from test anxiety. These bodily changes can include the following:

Perspiring
Sweaty palms
Wet, trembling hands
Nausea
Dry mouth
A knot in the stomach
Headache
Faintness
Muscle tension
Aching shoulders, back and neck
Rapid heart beat
Feeling too hot/cold

To recognize the sensation of test anxiety, a test-taker should monitor him/herself for the following sensations:

The physical distress symptoms as listed above
Emotional sensitivity, expressing emotional feelings such as the need to cry or laugh too much, or a sensation of anger or helplessness
A decreased ability to think, causing the test-taker to blank out or have racing thoughts that are hard to organize or control.

Though most students will feel some level of anxiety when faced with a test or exam, the majority can cope with that anxiety and maintain it at a manageable level. However, those who cannot are faced with a very real and very serious condition, which can and should be controlled for the immeasurable benefit of this sufferer.

Naturally, these sensations lead to negative results for the testing experience. The most common effects of test anxiety have to do with nervousness and mental blocking.

Nervousness

Nervousness can appear in several different levels:

The test-taker's difficulty, or even inability to read and understand the questions on the test
The difficulty or inability to organize thoughts to a coherent form
The difficulty or inability to recall key words and concepts relating to the testing questions (especially essays)
The receipt of poor grades on a test, though the test material was well known by the test taker

Conversely, a person may also experience mental blocking, which involves:

Blanking out on test questions
Only remembering the correct answers to the questions when the test has already finished.

Fortunately for test anxiety sufferers, beating these feelings, to a large degree, has to do with proper preparation. When a test taker has a feeling of preparedness, then anxiety will be dramatically lessened.

The first step to resolving anxiety issues is to distinguish which of the two types of anxiety are being suffered. If the anxiety is a direct result of a lack of preparation, this should be considered a normal reaction, and the anxiety level (as opposed to the test results) shouldn't be anything to worry about. However, if, when adequately prepared, the test-taker still panics, blanks out, or seems to overreact, this is not a fully rational reaction. While this can be considered normal too, there are many ways to combat and overcome these effects.

Remember that anxiety cannot be entirely eliminated, however, there are ways to minimize it, to make the anxiety easier to manage. Preparation is one of the best ways to minimize test anxiety. Therefore the following techniques are wise in order to best fight off any anxiety that may want to build.

To begin with, try to avoid cramming before a test, whenever it is possible. By trying to memorize an entire term's worth of information in one day, you'll be shocking your system, and not giving yourself a very good chance to absorb the information. This is an easy path to anxiety, so for those who suffer from test anxiety, cramming should not even be considered an option.

Instead of cramming, work throughout the semester to combine all of the material which is presented throughout the semester, and work on it gradually as the course goes by, making sure to master the main concepts first, leaving minor details for a week or so before the test.

To study for the upcoming exam, be sure to pose questions that may be on the examination, to gauge the ability to answer them by integrating the ideas from your texts, notes and lectures, as well as any supplementary readings.

If it is truly impossible to cover all of the information that was covered in that particular term, concentrate on the most important portions, that can be covered very well. Learn these concepts as best as possible, so that when the test comes, a goal can be made to use these concepts as presentations of your knowledge.

In addition to study habits, changes in attitude are critical to beating a struggle with test anxiety. In fact, an improvement of the perspective over the entire test-taking experience can actually help a test taker to enjoy studying and therefore improve the overall experience. Be certain not to overemphasize the significance of the grade - know that the result of the test is neither a reflection of self worth, nor is it a measure of intelligence; one grade will not predict a person's future success.

To improve an overall testing outlook, the following steps should be tried:

Keeping in mind that the most reasonable expectation for taking a test is to expect to try to demonstrate as much of what you know as you possibly can.
Reminding ourselves that a test is only one test; this is not the only one, and there will be others.
The thought of thinking of oneself in an irrational, all-or-nothing term should be avoided at all costs.
A reward should be designated for after the test, so there's something to look forward to. Whether it be going to a movie, going out to eat, or simply visiting friends, schedule it in advance, and do it no matter what result is expected on the exam.

Test-takers should also keep in mind that the basics are some of the most important things, even beyond anti-anxiety techniques and studying. Never neglect the basic social, emotional and biological needs, in order to try to absorb information. In order to best achieve, these three factors must be held as just as important as the studying itself.

Study Steps

Remember the following important steps for studying:

Maintain healthy nutrition and exercise habits. Continue both your recreational activities and social pass times. These both contribute to your physical and emotional well being.
Be certain to get a good amount of sleep, especially the night before the test, because when you're overtired you are not able to perform to the best of your best ability.
Keep the studying pace to a moderate level by taking breaks when they are needed, and varying the work whenever possible, to keep the mind fresh instead of getting bored.
When enough studying has been done that all the material that can be learned has been learned, and the test taker is prepared for the test, stop studying and do something relaxing such as listening to music, watching a movie, or taking a warm bubble bath.

There are also many other techniques to minimize the uneasiness or apprehension that is experienced along with test anxiety before, during, or even after the examination. In fact, there are a great deal of things that can be done to stop anxiety from interfering with lifestyle and performance. Again, remember that anxiety will not be eliminated entirely, and it shouldn't be. Otherwise that "up" feeling for exams would not exist, and most of us depend on that sensation to perform better than usual. However, this anxiety has to be at a level that is manageable.

Of course, as we have just discussed, being prepared for the exam is half the battle right away. Attending all classes, finding out what knowledge will be expected on the exam, and knowing the exam schedules are easy steps to lowering anxiety. Keeping up with work will remove the need to cram, and efficient study habits will eliminate wasted time. Studying should be done in an ideal location for concentration, so that it is simple to become interested in the material and give it complete attention. A method such as SQ3R (Survey, Question, Read, Recite, Review) is a wonderful key to follow to make sure that the study habits are as effective as possible, especially in the case of learning from a textbook. Flashcards are great techniques for memorization. Learning to take good notes will mean that notes will be full of useful information, so that less sifting will need to be done to seek out what is pertinent for studying. Reviewing notes after class and then again on occasion will keep the information fresh in the mind. From notes that have been taken summary sheets and outlines can be made for simpler reviewing.

A study group can also be a very motivational and helpful place to study, as there will be a sharing of ideas, all of the minds can work together, to make sure that everyone understands, and the studying will be made more interesting because it will be a social occasion.

Basically, though, as long as the test-taker remains organized and self confident, with efficient study habits, less time will need to be spent studying, and higher grades will be achieved.

To become self confident, there are many useful steps. The first of these is "self talk." It has been shown through extensive research, that self-talk for students who suffer from test anxiety, should be well monitored, in order to make sure that it contributes to self confidence as opposed to sinking the student. Frequently the self talk of test-anxious students is negative or self-defeating, thinking that everyone else is smarter and faster, that they always mess up, and that if they don't do well, they'll fail the entire course. It is important to decreasing anxiety that awareness is made of self talk. Try writing any negative self thoughts and then disputing them with a positive statement instead. Begin self-encouragement as though it was a friend speaking. Repeat positive statements to help reprogram the mind to believing in successes instead of failures.

Helpful Techniques

Other extremely helpful techniques include:

Self-visualization of doing well and reaching goals
While aiming for an "A" level of understanding, don't try to "overprotect" by setting your expectations lower. This will only convince the mind to stop studying in order to meet the lower expectations.
Don't make comparisons with the results or habits of other students. These are individual factors, and different things work for different people, causing different results.
Strive to become an expert in learning what works well, and what can be done in order to improve. Consider collecting this data in a journal.
Create rewards for after studying instead of doing things before studying that will only turn into avoidance behaviors.
Make a practice of relaxing - by using methods such as progressive relaxation, self-hypnosis, guided imagery, etc - in order to make relaxation an automatic sensation.
Work on creating a state of relaxed concentration so that concentrating will take on the focus of the mind, so that none will be wasted on worrying.
Take good care of the physical self by eating well and getting enough sleep.
Plan in time for exercise and stick to this plan.

Beyond these techniques, there are other methods to be used before, during and after the test that will help the test-taker perform well in addition to overcoming anxiety.

Before the exam comes the academic preparation. This involves establishing a study schedule and beginning at least one week before the actual date of the test. By doing this, the anxiety of not having enough time to study for the test will be automatically eliminated. Moreover, this will make the studying a much more effective experience, ensuring that the learning will be an easier process. This relieves much undue pressure on the test-taker.

Summary sheets, note cards, and flash cards with the main concepts and examples of these main concepts should be prepared in advance of the actual studying time. A topic should never be eliminated from this process. By omitting a topic because it isn't expected to be on the test is only setting up the test-taker for anxiety should it actually appear on the exam. Utilize the course syllabus for laying out the topics that should be studied. Carefully go over the notes that were made in class, paying special attention to any of the issues that the professor took special care to emphasize while lecturing in class. In the textbooks, use the chapter review, or if possible, the chapter tests, to begin your review.

It may even be possible to ask the instructor what information will be covered on the exam, or what the format of the exam will be (for example, multiple choice, essay, free form, true-false). Additionally, see if it is possible to find out how many questions will be on the test. If a review sheet or sample test has been offered by the professor, make good use of it, above anything else, for the preparation for the test. Another great resource for getting to know the examination is reviewing tests from previous semesters. Use these tests to review, and aim to achieve a 100% score on each of the possible topics. With a few exceptions, the goal that you set for yourself is the highest one that you will reach.

Take all of the questions that were assigned as homework, and rework them to any other possible course material. The more problems reworked, the more skill and confidence will form as a result. When forming the solution to a problem, write out each of the steps. Don't simply do head work. By doing as many steps on paper as possible, much clarification and therefore confidence will be formed. Do this with as many homework problems as possible, before checking the answers. By checking the answer after each problem, a reinforcement will exist, that will not be on the exam. Study situations should be as exam-like as possible, to prime the test-taker's system for the experience. By waiting to check the answers at the end, a psychological advantage will be formed, to decrease the stress factor.

Another fantastic reason for not cramming is the avoidance of confusion in concepts, especially when it comes to mathematics. 8-10 hours of study will become one hundred percent more effective if it is spread out over a week or at least several days, instead of doing it all in one sitting. Recognize that the human brain requires time in order to assimilate new material, so frequent breaks and a span of study time over several days will be much more beneficial.

Additionally, don't study right up until the point of the exam. Studying should stop a minimum of one hour before the exam begins. This allows the brain to rest and put things in their proper order. This will also provide the time to become as relaxed as possible when going into the examination room. The test-taker will also have time to eat well and eat sensibly. Know that the brain needs food as much as the rest of the body. With enough food and enough sleep, as well as a relaxed attitude, the body and the mind are primed for success.

Avoid any anxious classmates who are talking about the exam. These students only spread anxiety, and are not worth sharing the anxious sentimentalities.

Before the test also involves creating a positive attitude, so mental preparation should also be a point of concentration. There are many keys to creating a positive attitude. Should fears become rushing in, make a visualization of taking the exam, doing well, and seeing an A written on the paper. Write out a list of affirmations that will bring a feeling of confidence, such as "I am doing well in my English class," "I studied well and know my material," "I enjoy this class." Even if the affirmations aren't believed at first, it sends a positive message to the subconscious which will result in an alteration of the overall belief system, which is the system that creates reality.

If a sensation of panic begins, work with the fear and imagine the very worst! Work through the entire scenario of not passing the test, failing the entire course, and dropping out of school, followed by not getting a job, and pushing a shopping cart through the dark alley where you'll live. This will place things into perspective! Then, practice deep breathing and create a visualization of the opposite situation - achieving an "A" on the exam, passing the entire course, receiving the degree at a graduation ceremony.

On the day of the test, there are many things to be done to ensure the best results, as well as the most calm outlook. The following stages are suggested in order to maximize test-taking potential:

Begin the examination day with a moderate breakfast, and avoid any coffee or beverages with caffeine if the test taker is prone to jitters. Even people who are used to managing caffeine can feel jittery or light-headed when it is taken on a test day.
Attempt to do something that is relaxing before the examination begins. As last minute cramming clouds the mastering of overall concepts, it is better to use this time to create a calming outlook.
Be certain to arrive at the test location well in advance, in order to provide time to select a location that is away from doors, windows and other distractions, as well as giving enough time to relax before the test begins.
Keep away from anxiety generating classmates who will upset the sensation of stability and relaxation that is being attempted before the exam.
Should the waiting period before the exam begins cause anxiety, create a self-distraction by reading a light magazine or something else that is relaxing and simple.

During the exam itself, read the entire exam from beginning to end, and find out how much time should be allotted to each individual problem. Once writing the exam, should more time be taken for a problem, it should be abandoned, in order to begin another problem. If there is time at the end, the unfinished problem can always be returned to and completed.

Read the instructions very carefully - twice - so that unpleasant surprises won't follow during or after the exam has ended.

When writing the exam, pretend that the situation is actually simply the completion of homework within a library, or at home. This will assist in forming a relaxed atmosphere, and will allow the brain extra focus for the complex thinking function.

Begin the exam with all of the questions with which the most confidence is felt. This will build the confidence level regarding the entire exam and will begin a quality momentum. This will also create encouragement for trying the problems where uncertainty resides.

Going with the "gut instinct" is always the way to go when solving a problem. Second guessing should be avoided at all costs. Have confidence in the ability to do well.

For essay questions, create an outline in advance that will keep the mind organized and make certain that all of the points are remembered. For multiple choice, read every answer, even if the correct one has been spotted - a better one may exist.

Continue at a pace that is reasonable and not rushed, in order to be able to work carefully. Provide enough time to go over the answers at the end, to check for small errors that can be corrected.

Should a feeling of panic begin, breathe deeply, and think of the feeling of the body releasing sand through its pores. Visualize a calm, peaceful place, and include all of the sights, sounds and sensations of this image. Continue the deep breathing, and take a few minutes to continue this with closed eyes. When all is well again, return to the test.

If a "blanking" occurs for a certain question, skip it and move on to the next question. There will be time to return to the other question later. Get everything done that can be done, first, to guarantee all the grades that can be compiled, and to build all of the confidence possible. Then return to the weaker questions to build the marks from there.

Remember, one's own reality can be created, so as long as the belief is there, success will follow. And remember: anxiety can happen later, right now, there's an exam to be written!

After the examination is complete, whether there is a feeling for a good grade or a bad grade, don't dwell on the exam, and be certain to follow through on the reward that was promised...and enjoy it! Don't dwell on any mistakes that have been made, as there is nothing that can be done at this point anyway.

Additionally, don't begin to study for the next test right away. Do something relaxing for a while, and let the mind relax and prepare itself to begin absorbing information again.

From the results of the exam - both the grade and the entire experience, be certain to learn from what has gone on. Perfect studying habits and work some more on confidence in order to make the next examination experience even better than the last one.

Learn to avoid places where openings occurred for laziness, procrastination and day dreaming.

Use the time between this exam and the next one to better learn to relax, even learning to relax on cue, so that any anxiety can be controlled during the next exam. Learn how to relax the body. Slouch in your chair if that helps. Tighten and then relax all of the different muscle groups, one group at a time, beginning with the feet and then working all the way up to the neck and face. This will ultimately relax the muscles more than they were to begin with. Learn how to breathe deeply and comfortably, and focus on this breathing going in and out as a relaxing thought. With every exhale, repeat the word "relax."

As common as test anxiety is, it is very possible to overcome it. Make yourself one of the test-takers who overcome this frustrating hindrance.

Special Report: Additional Bonus Material

Due to our efforts to try to keep this book to a manageable length, we've created a link that will give you access to all of your additional bonus material.

Please visit http://www.mometrix.com/bonus948/chpn to access the information.

Made in the USA
Middletown, DE
09 February 2018